Study Guide for the
Generalist Hospice and
Palliative Nurse

Third Edition

Editor

Lynn Borstelmann, RN, MN, CHPN®, AOCN
Director, Oncology Services
The Nebraska Medical Center
Omaha, Nebraska

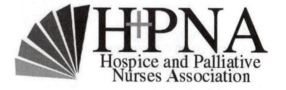

Hospice and Palliative
Nurses Association

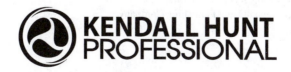

KENDALL HUNT
PROFESSIONAL

Development of this Study Guide

has been made possible by the

Hospice and Palliative Nurses Association

CONTENTS

CONTRIBUTORS

Patricia H. Berry, PhD, ACHPN®
Assistant Professor
University of Utah College of Nursing
Salt Lake City, UT

Lynn Borstelmann, RN, MN, CHPN®, AOCN (Editor)
Director, Oncology Services
The Nebraska Medical Center
Omaha, NE

Mary Ersek, PhD, RN
Research Scientist
Pain Research Department
Swedish Medical Center
Seattle, WA

Betty R. Ferrell, PhD, FAAN
Research Scientist
City of Hope National Medical Center
Duarte, CA

Marlene A.S. Foreman, BSN, MN, APRN-BC,
    ACHPN®
Clinical Nurse Specialist
Hospice of Acadiana
LaFayette, LA

Rose Anne Indelicato, MSN, ACHPN®, OCN
Program Manager: Pain Management and Palliative
    Care
Visiting Nurse Services in West Chester
White Plains, NY

Jeanne M. Martinez, RN, MPN, CHPN®
Quality and Education Specialist
Northwest Memorial Home Health Care
Chicago, IL

Judith A. Paice, PhD, RN, FAAN
Director Cancer Pain
Northwestern University
School of Medicine
Division of Hematology-Oncology
    Chicago, IL

Dena Jean Sutermaster, RN, MSN, CHPN®
Director of Education/Research
Hospice and Palliative Nurses Association
Pittsburgh, PA

CONTENT REVIEWERS

Patricia H. Berry, PhD, ACHPN®
Assistant Professor
University of Utah College of Nursing
Salt Lake City, UT

Sharmon Figenshaw, RN, MN, ARNP
Hospice/Palliative Nurse Practitioner
Providence Hospice and Home Care of Snohomish County
Everett, WA

Nancy L. Grandovic, RN, BSN, MEd.
Assistant Director of Education
Hospice and Palliative Nurses Association
Pittsburgh, PA

Karen A. Kehl, RN, MS, CHPN®
Research Assistant/On-call Nurse
University of Wisconsin-Madison
School of Nursing/HospiceCare, Inc.
Madison, WI

Candace A. Kinser, RN, CHPN®
Public Relations Director and Staff Nurse
Inspiration Hospice
Salt Lake City, UT

Fran Koubek, RN, MSN, CHPN®
Nurse Specialist
Hospice of Dayton
Dayton, OH

Judy Lentz, RN, MSN, NHA
CEO
Hospice and Palliative Nurses Association
Pittsburgh, PA

David J. Maxwell, RN, BSN, CHPN®
Staff Nurse
Marian Franciscan Center
Milwaukee, WI

Mary Lynn McPherson, PharmD, BCPS
Associate Professor
University of Maryland

School of Pharmacy
Hospice Consultant Pharmacist
Baltimore, MD

Annice O'Doherty, RN, CHPN®
Hospice Case Manager
Hospice of the Chesapeake
Annapolis, MD

Patricia Pollina, RN, BSN, CHPN®
Staff RN
Nathan Adelson Hospice
Las Vegas, NV

Sue Robertson, RN, PhD, MS
Part-time Faculty
California State University, Fullerton
Per Diem Staff Nurse
San Diego Hospice and Palliative Care
Fullerton, CA

Marilyn Smith-Stoner, RN, PhD, CHPN®
Assistant Professor
California State University Fullerton
Fullerton, CA

Pam Stephenson, RN, MSN, CHPN(R), AOCN, CS
Clinical Nurse Specialist
Forum Health-Cancer Care Centers
Youngstown, OH

Dena Jean Sutermaster, RN, MSN, CHPN®
Director of Education/Research
Hospice and Palliative Nurses Association
Pittsburgh, PA

Glenn Townsend, RN, BSN
Registered Nurse
St. Josephs Hospital
Phoenix, AZ

DISCLAIMER

The Hospice and Palliative Nurses Association, its officers and directors and the authors and reviewers of this Study Guide make no claims that buying or studying it will guarantee a passing score on the CHPN® Certification examination.

EDITOR'S COMMENTS/INTRODUCTION

My membership number in the Hospice and Palliative Nurses Association is 73. It has been my privilege to be a member and a participant in activities of the association since very early in its existence. At the time I joined, the organization lacked a dedicated office and staff, yet the nurses coming together to develop the association were incredibly committed to promoting and supporting the practice of hospice nursing. That commitment continues today as the organization continues to provide leadership in all areas of hospice and palliative nursing practice.

The *HPNA Study Guide for the Generalist Hospice and Palliative Nurse* and its companion, the *Core Curriculum for the Generalist Hospice and Palliative Nurse*, are valuable resources to nurses in assessing and expanding their knowledge of hospice and palliative nursing practice. These materials along with a wealth of literature—books, journals, websites, clinical guidelines, standards—that did not exist 25 years ago provide the basis for professional development in the practice with the goal of continuing to provide excellence in palliative care for patients and families facing life threatening illness. This edition of the Study Guide provides nurses with review materials in the form of questions, case studies, and medication calculations and incorporates items used in the End-Of-Life Nursing Education Consortium (ELNEC) curriculum (with permission).It divides questions in general categories similar to chapters in the *Core Curriculum*, which should enable the nurse to focus on specific areas where study or review are needed. The *Study Guide* provides a wide range of material in all aspects of hospice and palliative nursing practice. I am grateful to the many nurses who provided items and reviewed items to ensure that the material will be valuable to the learner and relevant to clinical practice.

I would like to dedicate my work on this *Study Guide* to my mother and my aunt, both of whom have benefited from the expertise of hospice and palliative nurses since the 2nd edition was published. We all want the best for our families and communities, and that means nurses who are knowledgeable in hospice and palliative practice. This *Study Guide* provides nurses dedicated to this specialty a resource to support their continuing education and development.

I am grateful for having had the opportunity to support this project and appreciate the confidence of Judy Lentz, HPNA CEO, Dena Jean Sutermaster, HPNA Director of Education/Research, and Patricia H. Berry, editor of the Core Curriculum. I would also like to thank Amy Killmeyer, HPNA Office Manager, and the National Office staff for their assistance in putting the *Study Guide* together. I challenge all of you using this Study Guide to participate in HPNA in whatever way you can—in my opinion you will gain much more professionally from the experience than you hope to give.

Lynn Borstelmann, RN, MN, CHPN®, AOCN, NEA-BC
Director, Oncology Services
The Nebraska Medical Center
Omaha, Nebraska

Study Questions
and Answers

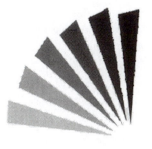

Overview and Care Setting

1. The nurse is orienting a new staff member on a unit that cares for many patients at the end of life. Which comment by the nurse correctly reflects a principle of palliative care?

    A. "We're busy because most people prefer to die in a hospital rather than at home where they would be a burden."

    B. "Death and dying are not discussed much here in order to maintain hope for patients and families."

    C. "Because our patients often are uncomfortable, they need physical care more than psychological or spiritual care."

    D. "Patients are eligible for palliative care even though they are also receiving curative treatment."

2. Which of the following was the first hospice in the United States?

    A. Memorial Sloan Kettering Hospice in New York City

    B. Hospice of the Western Reserve in Cleveland

    C. St. Joseph's Hospice in Boston

    D. The Connecticut Hospice in New Haven

3. The difference between the origin of hospice and palliative care in the United States is

    A. The hospice movement was part of the establishment

    B. The hospice movement was part of hospital sponsored programs

    C. Palliative care grew from academic, teaching hospitals

    D. Palliative care movement grew from a grassroots movement

1. Answer is D

    A. Incorrect: This is not a true statement; most people state that they would prefer to die in the comfort and familiarity of their own home.

    B. Incorrect: Palliative care provides support to patients and families facing advanced, life-threatening illness. Issues and concerns regarding death and dying are discussed with patients and families while maintaining realistic hope for quality of life and the time remaining for the patient.

    C. Incorrect: While patients need physical care they need that care in the context of comprehensive care, which includes attention to psychological and spiritual needs at the end of life.

    D. **Correct**: Palliative care does not limit a patient's options to pursue curative treatment but enhances the patient's quality of life by maximizing supportive care.

2. Answer is D

    A. Incorrect: Memorial Sloan Kettering is a cancer hospital.

    B. Incorrect: Hospice of the Western Reserve opened at a later time.

    C. Incorrect: St. Joseph's Hospice is located in London and was the name of the early hospice opened by Dame Cicely Saunders, the founder of the hospice movement.

    D. **Correct**: The Connecticut Hospice was founded by Florence Wald (former Dean of the Yale Nursing School) in the early 1970s.

3. Answer is C

    A. Incorrect: Hospice was introduced in the 1970s replicating a movement initiated in England and was a grassroots movement to change and improve care of the dying.

    B. Incorrect: The hospice movement was a national movement not a hospital-sponsored program.

    C. **Correct**: Palliative care units originated in the academic teaching hospitals as demonstration projects. The focus has been to move the philosophy of hospice upstream to encourage the application of the philosophy earlier in the disease trajectory and to allow patients a choice of therapies.

    D. Incorrect: Palliative care did not grow out of a grassroots movement.

4. Which of the following is the best description of hospice?

    A. A type of care utilized when nothing more can be done for the patient

    B. A philosophy of care to improve quality of life for the terminally ill

    C. A place where people are sent to die

    D. Available to patients and families only if the patient is at home

5. When comparing eligibility for hospice care versus palliative care, which of the following is true?

    A. Palliative care allows for more aggressive therapies

    B. Both have federal guidelines for enrollment

    C. Palliative care is not holistic

    D. Hospice has a broader enrollment

6. The eligibility for hospice and palliative care is

    A. Six month prognosis for both

    B. Six month prognosis for hospice and no time limit for palliative care

    C. Not affected by prognosis

    D. Not affected by time limits

4. Answer is B

    A. Incorrect: Hospice offers symptom management, physical care, emotional care, psychosocial care, spiritual care and bereavement care. Much is done to improve the quality of life for the individual and their family.

    B. **Correct**: Hospice is truly a philosophy to improve quality of life for the terminally ill.

    C. Incorrect: Hospice is not a building although often there are inpatient hospice units/beds available for respite and for acute symptom management.

    D. Incorrect: Hospice care may be provided in residential settings other than the patient's home.

5. Answer is A

    A. **Correct**: Palliative care includes whatever therapies are medically indicated and desired by the patient.

    B. Incorrect: Palliative care does not have enrollment guidelines and is not formalized in a Medicare or Medicaid benefit like hospice care. However, some private insurers may have coverage for palliative care and it may be defined within an individual health insurance plan or policy.

    C. Incorrect: Palliative care is intended to include multiple dimensions of care like hospice although programs may vary and there is no standard benefit as with hospice care.

    D. Incorrect: Hospice care covers the final six months of life—palliative care can cover a much longer period depending on the disease.

6. Answer is B

    A. Incorrect: Eligibility for palliative care exceeds six months especially in diseases such as Alzheimer's.

    B. **Correct**: Although hospice has a requirement for certification by the physician of a six-month prognosis, palliative care does not have this requirement.

    C. Incorrect: Eligibility for hospice care is directly related to prognosis.

    D. Incorrect: Eligibility for hospice is directly related to time limit of six months if the disease runs its natural course.

7. When is aggressive treatment **NOT** indicated?

   A. Cure is possible

   B. There is a realistic chance of worthwhile prolongation of life

   C. The side effects of the treatment are more distressing than the potential benefits

   D. A patient chooses a clinical trial with informed consent

8. Currently, palliative care is primarily delivered in which of the following settings?

   A. Home

   B. Acute care setting

   C. Nursing home

   D. Rehab setting

9. The nurse is having a discussion about barriers to quality end-of-life care with a co-worker. Which comment by the co-worker indicates misunderstanding and the need for more information?

   A. "A significant obstacle is healthcare professionals' lack of education about end-of-life care."

   B. "One reason people don't seek palliative care is that they are reluctant to give up hope."

   C. "The failure of healthcare professions to acknowledge the limits of traditional medicine is a major barrier."

   D. "It's essential to know someone has six months or less to live for end-of-life care to be started."

7. Answer is C

   A. Incorrect: When cure is possible, aggressive curative treatments are appropriate.

   B. Incorrect: It is appropriate to plan aggressive life-prolonging treatment when there is a realistic chance of worthwhile prolongation of life.

   C. **Correct**: It is inappropriate to plan aggressive curative treatment when the side effects of the treatment are more distressing than the potential benefits.

   D. Incorrect: It is appropriate to plan aggressive experimental treatment when a patient chooses a clinical trial with informed consent.

8. Answer is B

   A. Incorrect: Palliative care is currently delivered primarily in acute care settings. Palliative care in the home in the final six months is usually hospice care.

   B. **Correct**: Palliative care is currently delivered primarily in the acute care settings either in a dedicated unit or through palliative care consult teams.

   C. Incorrect: Although nursing homes are perfect for the delivery of palliative care, the movement has not penetrated this setting very far.

   D. Incorrect: Palliative care is inappropriate for rehab settings unless the patient has a life limiting progressively deteriorating disease.

9. Answer is D

   A. Incorrect: This is a true statement and indicates understanding.

   B. Incorrect: See A

   C. Incorrect: See A

   D. **Correct**: Quality end-of-life care should be initiated at the point in the illness when supportive care needs and concerns with quality of life become primary.

10. The nurse is developing the content for an interdisciplinary discussion on the concept of healing. Which statement should be included? Healing

   A. Is a medical outcome and is most appropriately directed by physicians

   B. Can occur only after the client's spiritual issues have been resolved with a chaplain

   C. Is possible if attention is paid to the multiple dimensions that influence a person's quality of life

   D. Occurs when the patient and family realize and accept that cure is not possible

11. The nurse is discussing aspects of suffering with the wife of a client. The client is dying from complications related to acquired immune deficiency syndrome (AIDS). Which statement by the nurse indicates understanding of the concept of suffering?

   A. "Suffering comes from many physical and psychological causes."

   B. "Suffering leads to finding a deeper meaning in life."

   C. "You will be able to determine what is causing your husband's suffering."

   D. "Your husband's suffering is related to the amount of pain he experiences."

12. Patients near the end of life most often fear

   A. Death itself and not finishing tasks

   B. Pain and being a burden to family

   C. Altered body image and not knowing what to expect

   D. Losing control and use of life-sustaining technology

10. Answer is C

   A. Incorrect: Healing is a process that includes all dimensions—physical, psychological and spiritual.

   B. Incorrect: Spiritual healing does not require the assistance of a chaplain although a spiritual advisor or counselor can certainly support the healing process.

   C. **Correct**: Healing can be promoted through the relationship of the healer and healed in addressing multiple dimensions of the person's quality of life.

   D. Incorrect: While this realization may help the patient and family be more open to other dimensions of healing, healing is still possible without this acceptance.

11. Answer is A

   A. **Correct**: There are multiple dimensions of suffering and suffering must be addressed from a comprehensive, holistic perspective.

   B. Incorrect: While finding a path through suffering and beyond can provide meaning for some people, suffering in and of itself does not provide deeper meaning. Families or patients could find this statement insensitive.

   C. Incorrect: It is not always possible to determine the source of suffering although a holistic assessment can help.

   D. Incorrect: Suffering has emotional and spiritual dimensions as well as physical. Nursing and hospice care should address all of the dimensions although this will not always be successful.

12. Answer is B

   A. Incorrect: The most common fears at the end of life include pain, fear of being a burden, fear of loss of control and independence and fear of dying alone.

   B. **Correct**: Both pain and being a burden to family are common fears of the dying.

   C. Incorrect: See A

   D. Incorrect: Losing control is a common fear, but both of these are not common fears.

13. Which statement is most accurate about suffering? Suffering

    A. Is a physical concept primarily concerned with pain and its prompt and continuous relief

    B. Involves the whole person and transcends the bio-psycho-social-spiritual dimension

    C. Is relatively easily recognized and interpreted by loved ones who know the patient well

    D. Can be diminished for the patient if the staff continues to focus on curing the disease

14. In order to improve the quality of end-of-life care in the clinical environment, the nurse should do all of the following **EXCEPT**

    A. Strive to make transfers of clients less frequent and less disruptive

    B. Create standardized protocols and outcome measures for this population

    C. Ensure continuity of care across time and provider settings

    D. Delay referral to hospice to maintain the patient's primary care

15. In caring for patients with life-threatening illnesses, the nurse must be aware of healthcare trends that impact end-of-life care. Which is a current trend in end-of-life care?

    A. Populations such as the uninsured and elderly enjoy equitable access to end-of-life care through public assistance programs

    B. End-of-life care programs have unrestricted eligibility and few rules for admission by those who need these services

    C. The healthcare team often delays referrals of patients to hospice and palliative care services until late in the illness

    D. Health insurance plans are legally prohibited from declining new enrollees who are in poor health and require end-of-life care

13. Answer is B

    A. Incorrect: Suffering is multidimensional and involves emotional and spiritual aspects as well as physical.

    B. **Correct**: This statement accurately reflects the multidimensional nature of suffering.

    C. Incorrect: Suffering can be multifaceted and complex and may require astute observation and presence. Different disciplinary perspectives in assessment can be of benefit.

    D. Incorrect: Suffering can be the result of multiple losses and other emotional/spiritual issues. By not addressing these real issues, suffering may be increased rather than diminished.

14. Answer is D

    A. Incorrect: This would be an appropriate action to provide continuity of care and quality care.

    B. Incorrect: Standardized protocols and outcome measures can help ensure that standards of care are met or exceeded.

    C. Incorrect: Ensuring continuity of care across time and provider settings is important in maintaining quality of care for the patient.

    D. **Correct**: Delaying referral to hospice to maintain the patient's primary care does not help improve quality end-of-life care, in fact it may diminish it. Hospice care is specialty end-of-life care; by denying access to hospice you are denying the patient specialized end-of-life care. Most hospices will partner with the primary care providers in developing an appropriate treatment plan that recognizes the patient's unique history.

15. Answer is C

    A. Incorrect: While the elderly are entitled to hospice services through the Hospice Medicare Benefit and can access palliative care services with Medicare coverage, the uninsured generally do not enjoy equal access to any healthcare services.

    B. Incorrect: Hospice programs have admission criteria and patients receiving care covered by the Medicare Hospice Benefit must meet certain criteria and have diagnosis and prognosis certified by a physician.

    C. **Correct**: For a variety of reasons, the healthcare team does delay referrals to hospice and palliative care services until late in the illness.

    D. Incorrect: Access to insurance may be limited by pre-existing condition provisions.

16. The nurse is caring for a terminally ill client who wishes to be discharged so that he can die at home. When planning for the discharge of this client with the interdisciplinary team, it is important to consider costs of care. The nurse understands that for a family caring for a dying patient at home

A. Costs of care can exhaust a family's financial resources

B. Medicare will cover all the older client's medical expenses

C. Services are readily available to allow the client to stay at home

D. Medicaid will be the primary provider of services

17. The nurse who wants to make changes in the healthcare system in end-of-life care realizes that it is important to

A. Become knowledgeable about system shortcomings in order to develop commitment to change

B. Concentrate on care that focuses on life-prolonging therapies rather than those that shorten life expectancy

C. Ask management to identify the primary aim of end-of-life care for the patient care team to implement

D. Realize that efforts towards system change are not in the scope of nursing practice

18. An example of advocacy in hospice and palliative care is

A. Testifying about the importance of quality terminal care

B. Negotiating continuous care reimbursement with a private insurance company

C. Contacting an airline to get reduced airfare for distant family members

D. All of the above

16.   Answer is A

A.   **Correct**: The cost of medical care is a major factor in bankruptcy nationwide. The costs of caring for a patient at home may include lost income while having a role as a caregiver.

B.   Incorrect: Medicare coverage has limits on coverage and may include co-pays, coinsurance, and deductibles for various types of services.

C.   Incorrect: Services may not be available or affordable for personal caregiving and other basic needs even if costs of home health or hospice care are covered by insurance.

D.   Incorrect: Medicaid is a payer for care for the medically indigent, not a provider of services.

17.   Answer is A

A.   **Correct**: Understanding the current system and history will lead to more effective efforts for change.

B.   Incorrect: This would be counter to the goal of improving end-of-life care.

C.   Incorrect: This would not impact the system, only the patients cared for by that team.

D.   Incorrect: Nurses are an important voice in changing and improving healthcare in their role as advocates for populations of patients.

18.   Answer is D

A.   Incorrect: All the choices listed are examples of advocacy.

B.   Incorrect: All the choices listed are examples of advocacy.

C.   Incorrect: All the choices listed are examples of advocacy.

D.   **Correct**: This is the correct answer since all the choices listed are examples of advocacy. Advocacy is considered an important component of professional nursing practice.

19. An appropriate criterion for deciding to institute any given therapy for a terminally ill patient is if

   A. The potential benefits outweigh the potential risks or burdens to the patient

   B. The physician wants to try once more for a cure

   C. The family demands it

   D. It will prolong life

20. What is a therapeutic intervention that can be provided by any hospice team member to a suffering patient at the end of life?

   A. Sedation

   B. Massage therapy

   C. Hypnosis

   D. Presence

Interdisciplinary Team

21. Which factor places a new hospice nurse at risk for an increased emotional response to a client's death?

   A. Lack of home care experience

   B. The loss of a loved one within the past year

   C. Frequency of death experienced in the hospice setting

   D. Experience with clients who have advanced diseases

19.   Answer is A

    A. **Correct**: If the potential benefits outweigh the potential risk or burden to the patient, therapy should be instituted with permission of the patient.

    B. Incorrect: It is inappropriate for the physician to try once more for a cure in the terminally ill patient where cure is not achievable.

    C. Incorrect: The patient is the center of decision-making. Decisions to initiate therapies should not be done in response to the demands of the family.

    D. Incorrect: The decision to institute therapy should be in accordance with the patient's wishes and according to the plan of care. Prolongation of life is not necessarily providing quality of life, which should be the primary goal.

20.   Answer is D

    A. Incorrect: Sedation can only be ordered by a physician and administered by nursing professionals or family caregivers who have been taught.

    B. Incorrect: Massage therapy should be provided by a trained therapist.

    C. Incorrect: Hypnosis requires special skills.

    D. **Correct**: Care at the end of life can be frustrating when attempts to decrease suffering are either not possible or not successful. "Presence" is a way of expressing compassionate caring when actions are ineffective. Therapeutic presence can be a wonderful gift for patients and families.

Interdisciplinary Team

21.   Answer is B

    A. Incorrect: Lack of home care experience can be affected by training and skill development but does not affect emotional response.

    B. **Correct**: A nurse who is grieving herself may be at risk for an increased emotional response to a client's death, especially if the grief is not resolving.

    C. Incorrect: While frequency of death may be a factor in an increased emotional response by a nurse, this question is specifically asking about a new hospice nurse who presumably hasn't experienced frequent deaths yet.

    D. Incorrect: Experience with clients with advanced disease should assist the nurse in adjusting to caring for patients at the end of life.

22.   What is the primary benefit of interdisciplinary teamwork in end-of-life care?

    A. The patient and family do not have to make all the decisions

    B. Disciplines develop shared goals based on patient/family wishes

    C. The nurse is able to focus more on nursing issues for the patient

    D. Each discipline can create appropriate and unique goals for the patient

23.   The nurse is part of a collaborative team providing end-of-life care. Which remark by another team member indicates the best understanding of culturally sensitive end-of-life care?

    A. "I ask the patient who he wants to include in conversations about his illness."

    B. "I hold the patient's hand and get physically close to her to show I care."

    C. "I can predict how members of a particular ethnic group will respond to pain."

    D. "I feel it's our obligation to tell a patient bad news, even if the family objects."

24.   The nurse is part of an interdisciplinary team caring for an 11-year-old girl who has a malignant brain tumor. The parents have told the nurse that they prefer not to tell the child about her impending death and the nurse has shared this with the team. Several team members are frustrated about this situation and disagree with the parents' decision. What is the nurse's most appropriate response?

    A. Suggest that the physician tell the child so the parents don't have to

    B. Ask the hospital chaplain to talk with the family to offer them support

    C. Help the team members identify differing views on full disclosure

    D. Suggest that different team members care for this patient and family

22. Answer is B

    A. Incorrect: The goal is still to involve the patient and family in all decisions.

    B. **Correct**: Patient/family needs and preferences are assessed by different disciplines and a care plan is developed that meets the goals identified by the patient/family and team.

    C. Incorrect: While having a team does enable nursing to focus on nursing care, this is not the primary benefit of interdisciplinary teamwork.

    D. Incorrect: Separate goals would not provide coordinated care for the patient or family and would result in fragmentation.

23. Answer is A

    A. **Correct**: Culturally sensitive care implies assessments which determine the patient's needs and preferences.

    B. Incorrect: Personal space and the meaning of touch varies by cultural background and individual preference and actions should not be taken until an assessment is made.

    C. Incorrect: While response to pain may be influenced by cultural background, there are many other variables that affect an individual's response and assumptions should not be made without appropriate assessment.

    D. Incorrect: The degree of disclosure desired by a patient and family should be verified before proceeding.

24. Answer is C

    A. Incorrect: If the parents do not wish the child to be told about the impending death, the issue is not addressed by having the physician communicate against the parents' wishes.

    B. Incorrect: The parent's preferences do not necessarily indicate a need for a referral for a chaplain unless they requested such.

    C. **Correct**: Identifying differing views and rationale for such views may help the team try and see the parents' reactions from a different perspective.

    D. Incorrect: Team members should be able to handle differences that do not place a patient's safety in jeopardy.

25. The nurse is being oriented to palliative care. Which factor should the nurse identify as a requirement crucial to quality end-of-life care?

    A. Maintaining cost-effective analgesic protocols

    B. Using algorithms for symptom management

    C. Communicating effectively with clients and families

    D. Evaluating and measuring the outcomes of care

26. A nursing instructor is helping nursing students with clinical experience in a hospice facility. The faculty member and students are discussing ways the behavior of healthcare professionals can produce a communication barrier. Which statement by a nursing student would require the faculty member to follow up with the student?

    A. "I will complete a cultural assessment in order to understand the client's communication preferences."

    B. "I will keep an emotional distance in order to maintain a professional relationship with clients."

    C. "I may not always know the answers to questions that the client or family may ask."

    D. "I will ask my instructor to assist me if I am feeling uncomfortable in providing care."

27. The nurse is preparing a staff development conference on adaptive and maladaptive mechanisms clients and families use when dealing with the diagnosis of a life-threatening illness. What should the nurse use as an example of an adaptive behavior?

    A. Use of humor as a means to reduce stress

    B. Expressions of guilt by either patient or family

    C. A patient or family member exhibiting depression

    D. Use of denial over a prolonged period of time

25.   Answer is D

   A. Incorrect: Cost-effectiveness is a measure of efficiency, not quality.

   B. Incorrect: Algorithms may be a basis for quality care if they are evidenced-based and outcomes are measured, but are a process tool that does not guarantee quality.

   C. Incorrect: Good communication is a component of good quality of life care but if quality of care is not measured it cannot be determined if quality of care was provided or not.

   D. **Correct**: This is the best answer as evaluating and measuring the outcomes of care is critical to understanding whether the good communication, cost-effective and evidence-based care had the intended effect.

26.   Answer is B

   A. Incorrect: A cultural assessment would be an excellent foundation to understand communication preferences.

   B. **Correct**: The therapeutic use of self and creating a caring relationship are not consistent with emotional distance.

   C. Incorrect: This sentence demonstrates insight by the student on his/her limitations.

   D. Incorrect: This would be an appropriate response in seeking the instructor's support and guidance when there is discomfort.

27.   Answer is A

   A. **Correct**: Humor is a positive and adaptive response.

   B. Incorrect: Guilt can have a negative impact.

   C. Incorrect: Depression is not an adaptive response and requires assessment and treatment.

   D. Incorrect: While some denial may be adaptive, prolonged significant denial can be maladaptive.

28. The nurse is facilitating a staff discussion about myths and realities of communication in palliative care. Which is a correct statement about communication?

    A. "We can never give someone too much information."

    B. "We communicate only when we choose to communicate."

    C. "The majority of messages we send are non-verbal."

    D. "Communication is primarily words and their meanings."

29. Clients and families facing life-threatening illness expect that communication between themselves and a healthcare professional will include all of the following **EXCEPT:** The professional will

    A. Decide what client issues need to be addressed first

    B. Discuss the client's care with the healthcare team

    C. Be honest/truthful in all communications

    D. Be available to listen to a client's concerns

30. The nurse is talking with colleagues about the emotional challenges of working with dying patients and their families. The nurse identifies all of the following as appropriate responses to staff grief **EXCEPT**

    A. Helping plan a unit ceremony to honor all patients who have died recently

    B. Recognizing that personal grief should not be expressed by the nurse

    C. Seeking the support of a trusted colleague who has had similar experiences

    D. Consulting with a pastoral care worker or spiritual advisor for assistance

28.   Answer is C

     A. Incorrect: Patients and families can definitely be overwhelmed by too much information.

     B. Incorrect: Communication occurs at many levels and cannot always be controlled by the person sending the messages.

     C. **Correct**: As much as 80% of all communication may occur at the non-verbal level.

     D. Incorrect: See B

29.   Answer is A

     A. **Correct**: Clients and families expect to be able to develop a mutual plan of care with the team that respects their own needs and preferences.

     B. Incorrect: Clients and families expect that care will be discussed and coordinated with the other members of the healthcare team.

     C. Incorrect: Clients and families expect honesty and truthfulness in dealings with professionals.

     D. Incorrect: Clients and families do expect that they will be listened to and their needs will be attended to.

30.   Answer is B

     A. Incorrect: Ceremonies can help staff honor memories and grieve the losses inherent in their week.

     B. **Correct**: The nurse does experience loss in working with the dying and their families, grief is the emotional response to loss and needs to be expressed to facilitate adaptive coping.

     C. Incorrect: Social support from colleagues who understand the work and the losses is an appropriate response to grief.

     D. Incorrect: Consulting with spiritual care providers can be of benefit in responding to grief.

31. The nurse is facilitating the monthly bereavement support group for the hospice agency. Mr. C, whose wife of 14 years died five months ago, states "I still can't get through a week without crying sometimes. I know I should be at least starting to move on a bit." The best response by the nurse would be

    A. "Most people find it takes six months before things get back to normal."

    B. "It is still so soon after your wife's death, but you will be feeling better soon."

    C. "There is no way to predict when your grieving will be over."

    D. "Perhaps you would like to have individual counseling for more intensive therapy."

32. The nurse may experience feelings of anxiety and grief when caring for clients and families facing death and the dying process. In order for the nurse to be able to continue to provide quality care, it is important to obtain personal support by

    A. Seeking out the assistance of team members whenever necessary

    B. Periodic transfers to another unit to avoid caring for dying patients

    C. Maintaining an emotional distance from clients and families

    D. Scheduling counseling at regular intervals to deal with loss issues

33. Change in the healthcare system begins on the clinical unit. In order to improve end-of-life care within an agency, the nurse should do all of the following **EXCEPT**

    A. Develop outcome measures for improved end-of-life care against which to measure progress

    B. Ask physicians, as health team leaders, to direct the end-of-life care team and make system improvements

    C. Be conscious of end-of-life care financial costs and treatment burdens on patients and families

    D. Focus on quality end-of-life care so that death is a positive outcome rather than a treatment failure

31.   Answer is C

A. Incorrect: Since grief is individual, it would be incorrect to give this patient a specific timeframe, especially since he is still grieving at five months.

B. Incorrect: Like A, this answer is incorrect because it makes a prediction that may not be accurate.

C. **Correct**: This validates that there is not prediction and that is to be expected, making the client's experience normalized.

D. Incorrect: There is no indication of complicated or abnormal grieving requiring further intervention. The symptoms the client is experiencing are normal.

32.   Answer is A

A. **Correct**: One of the significant benefits of interdisciplinary teamwork is the support and assistance that colleagues can provide for each other.

B. Incorrect: Avoidance is not an adaptive response, although a break from caring for dying patients may be warranted at times.

C. Incorrect: Emotional distance does not allow the professional to appropriately use the self therapeutically in the relationship with the client and to provide a supportive, caring environment.

D. Incorrect: Counseling at regular intervals is not necessary although it may be of positive benefit for some.

33.   Answer is B

A. Incorrect: Outcome measures are critical for evaluating the quality of care.

B. **Correct**: Quality improvement is best directed by the people who do the work and understand the process and should involve all team members or representatives.

C. Incorrect: The team should be aware of the costs/benefits of care both financially and in terms of quality of life.

D. Incorrect: The goal of quality care and attending to the client's quality of life is important in improving end-of-life care.

34. An effective way to accelerate improvement of end-of-life care services is by utilizing rapid cycle quality improvement. The fundamental questions that need to be addressed include all of the following **EXCEPT**

   A. What are we trying to accomplish?

   B. How will we know that a change is an improvement?

   C. How many changes can we implement in the first year?

   D. What changes can we make that will result in improvement?

35. The purposes for attending the death of a hospice patient include all of the following **EXCEPT**

   A. Closure for hospice staff member

   B. Confirming the death

   C. Provision of comfort and support to the family

   D. Prompt removal of medical equipment and supplies

36. As a case manager, the hospice nurse

   A. Supervises the activities of the interdisciplinary team (IDT)

   B. Establishes the plan of care

   C. Coordinates and oversees the implementation of the IDT plan of care

   D. Directs the activities of the other members of the IDT

34. Answer is C

   A. Incorrect: This is an appropriate question to ask—what is our purpose/goal.

   B. Incorrect: This is an appropriate question to ask because it will lead us to measure our performance before and after changes are made.

   C. **Correct**: This is not a question that needs to be addressed because quantity of change is not the goal; rather the goal is to create meaningful changes that lead to measurable improvement.

   D. Incorrect: This is an appropriate question as it will help determine the changes that will be meaningful in producing the desired improvement.

35. Answer is D

   A. Incorrect: This is just one purpose.

   B. Incorrect: This is a second purpose.

   C. Incorrect: This is an additional purpose.

   D. **Correct**: This is not a purpose for attending the death of a hospice patient.

36. Answer is C

   A. Incorrect: The case manager is not administratively responsible for the team.

   B. Incorrect: The plan of care is the responsibility of the entire team not just the case manager.

   C. **Correct**: The case manager does in fact coordinate and oversee the implementation of the IDT plan of care.

   D. Incorrect: The interdisciplinary team is self directed. The case manager is an equal member of this team.

37. The palliative care patient's primary care physician

   A. Turns over the care of the patient to the palliative care service medical director upon admission

   B. Is responsible for the overall medical component of the palliative care program

   C. Usually continues to direct the medical care of the patient

   D. Is required to make home visits once the patient is discharged

38. Who must establish the initial hospice plan of care to reflect the Medicare guidelines?

   A. The nurse and social worker

   B. The IDT and attending physician

   C. The admitting nurse

   D. The nurse, social worker, and the chaplain

39. Interdisciplinary Collaborative Practice in the hospice setting includes

   A. The coordination of patient care for other healthcare providers

   B. Interaction with IDT members at time of admission

   C. The understanding that the nurse case manager makes all of the decisions regarding the patient's care

   D. The development of the plan of care in collaboration with the patient, family, other health and human service providers, and the IDT

40. Supervision of the nurse assistant includes

   A. Review of the care plan

   B. Observation of care being given and teaching an aspect of care

   C. Documentation of the supervisory visit

   D. All of the above

37. Answer is C

    A. Incorrect: The primary care physician does not turn the care of the patient over to the medical director of the palliative care service.

    B. Incorrect: The primary care physician is not responsible for the overall medical component of the palliative care program—this would be the responsibility of the medical director of the palliative care service.

    C. **Correct**: The primary care physician usually continues to direct the medical care of the patient.

    D. Incorrect: The primary care physician is not required to make home visits.

38. Answer is B

    A. Incorrect: All team members are responsible for the plan of care.

    B. **Correct**: The entire interdisciplinary team and the attending physician are responsible for establishing the hospice plan of care.

    C. Incorrect: All team members are responsible for the plan of care.

    D. Incorrect: All team members are responsible for the plan of care.

39. Answer is D

    A. Incorrect: This choice leaves out the family and patient and assumes coordination <u>for</u> rather than <u>with</u>.

    B. Incorrect: This choice leaves out the patient, family, other health and human service providers.

    C. Incorrect: Decision-making is not the responsibility of one individual.

    D. **Correct**: Interdisciplinary collaboration practice includes all involved in the case including patient, family, other health or human service providers and the IDT.

40. Answer is D

    A. Incorrect: Review of the care plan is just one aspect of supervision.

    B. Incorrect: Observation of care being given and teaching an aspect of care is another aspect of supervision along with review of the care plan.

    C. Incorrect: Documentation of the supervisory visit is part of the supervision but not exclusively so.

    D. **Correct**: All choices listed are part of the supervision of the nurse assistant.

The following situation pertains to questions 41 and 42

You have been caring for Mr. R for 4 weeks. He was diagnosed with colon cancer 4 years ago and came to hospice for relief of his symptoms of abdominal pain and loss of appetite. You visit once a week. The social worker and chaplain have had phone contact with the wife and daughter, but the patient and family have declined visits beyond the social worker's initial assessment visit. You review Mr. R's plan of care with the patient and his wife at each visit. The following changes have taken place in the past week.

Mr. R is more fatigued, spending more time in bed and is unable to bathe or feed himself. Mrs. R is also very tired because she is doing more of the physical care of her husband.

41.   What changes would you initiate in the plan of care that would improve quality of life for both patient and family?

    A. Provide services of a nurse assistant if patient/family receptive

    B. Counsel his wife on her need to rest

    C. Teach his wife how to give a bed bath and make an occupied bed

    D. Initiate a referral to the hospice physical therapist

42.   Knowing that these changes indicate deterioration of the patient's disease, how would you use the IDT to provide coordinated care?

    A. Arrange for equipment and supplies that will make the patient's ongoing care easier for the patient and family

    B. Request that the social worker and chaplain call the patient and wife again to offer support and to arrange a visit

    C. Update the plan of care after consulting the attending physician for orders

    D. Refer the wife to a contract agency for homemaker services

41.   Answer is A

    A. **Correct**: This change would be most beneficial for patient and family.

    B. Incorrect: Providing assistance will allow the wife to get needed rest.

    C. Incorrect: Teaching the wife how to make an occupied bed and how to give a bed bath are appropriate but would not be the most beneficial in this situation.

    D. Incorrect: Making a physical therapy referral would not be appropriate in this situation.

42.   Answer is B

    A. Incorrect: While this is an appropriate intervention, it does not show how to use the IDT to provide coordinated care.

    B. **Correct**: This action demonstrates the use of the IDT. While the patient and wife had refused these supports before, the fact that the patient's condition and needs have changed may lead to a change in acceptance and so they should be offered again.

    C. Incorrect: This does not show the team involvement in developing the care plan.

    D. Incorrect: While this may be an appropriate action, the IDT may be able to provide volunteer assistance.

43. The social worker on the team and you do not agree on an approach to a family. Your best response to this conflict would be to?

   A. Contact the physician for orders

   B. Suppress your frustration and anger to avoid conflict

   C. Go to your supervisor to have him/her resolve the conflict

   D. Work with the social worker directly to resolve the issue

44. Which of the following examples would demonstrate crossing of professional boundaries?

   A. Making cookies for a patient

   B. Going to a patient's birthday party and missing your own son's party

   C. Staying an extra half hour to talk to the wife, who is upset

   D. Praying with a patient who has requested it

45. Your hospice program is very short on nursing staff and the supervisor has requested you to work on your day off. You are very tired but feel committed to the program. What would be your best response in order to meet the needs of the program and take care of yourself?

   A. Let the supervisor know that you are exhausted and need a day off if at all possible

   B. Suggest the supervisor take care of the patients because you are not going to

   C. Do the extra day without saying anything, because it won't help anyway

   D. Throw your hands up in the air and storm out of the room without answering

43. Answer is D

    A. Incorrect: It would be inappropriate to contact the physician in this situation.

    B. Incorrect: This passive aggressive avoidance response will not help in resolving the issue.

    C. Incorrect: The issue should be discussed and resolved by the parties involved—the nurse and the social worker. The supervisor should not be involved unless direct resolution efforts fail.

    D. **Correct**: Working directly with the social worker would be the best approach.

44. Answer is B

    A. Incorrect: This activity would be within professional boundaries.

    B. **Correct**: This example would definitely overstep the professional boundaries of the caregiver.

    C. Incorrect: This activity would be well within one's professional boundaries.

    D. Incorrect: This activity would be within professional boundaries as long as the patient requested it as indicated.

45. Answer is A

    A. **Correct**: Professionalism requires open communication with your assigned supervisor. Expressing your concerns is important to maintaining open communications and trust. If you feel that your safety and/or the patient's are being placed in jeopardy, then you must communicate this directly.

    B. Incorrect: This response would be unprofessional and unacceptable.

    C. Incorrect: Effective open communications are necessary to maintain trust and effective management. The direct supervisor should appreciate open communication and honesty in his/her workforce.

    D. Incorrect: This behavior is unprofessional and unacceptable.

46. Why is nursing research important to palliative care and to hospice? To

    A. Meet requirements of the Joint Commission

    B. Find better ways to manage the symptoms of cancer and its treatment

    C. Ensure that physicians will agree with the researched protocols

    D. Enhance the art and science of palliative and hospice nursing and to improve end-of-life care

47. You have been assigned to a new nurse as his preceptor. The most important component of this role is

    A. To provide friendship

    B. Assist, evaluate, and provide guidance

    C. Tell the new nurse how to perform procedures

    D. Provide networking opportunities

48. The role of the professional on the IDT is

    A. Well defined and with specified boundaries

    B. Carried out totally independent of other disciplines

    C. A reflection of unique expertise that is integrated into a coordinated team approach

    D. Performed without personal involvement or emotional attachment

46. Answer is D

    A. Incorrect: The Joint Commission does not require research.

    B. Incorrect: Research will help to develop better symptom management but not all hospice and palliative care patients have a diagnosis of cancer.

    C. Incorrect: Research will not necessarily lead to physician agreement.

    D. **Correct**: Research does enhance the art and science of palliative and hospice nursing to improve end-of-life care. It is evidence-based outcomes that assure practice and treatment changes if recommendations have a scientific basis.

47. Answer is B

    A. Incorrect: Friendship is important to relationship building but it is not the most important component of this role.

    B. **Correct**: Precepting is assisting, evaluating and guiding the new nurse to assure they develop a level of comfort to function independently.

    C. Incorrect: Precepting should be facilitating and guiding the new nurse not telling them how to perform procedures.

    D. Incorrect: Networking occurs whenever new people meet one another but is independent of any precepting responsibilities.

48. Answer is C

    A. Incorrect: The roles of the professionals on the IDT are not well defined, nor do they have strict boundaries. Each member of the team is focused on the individual's plan of care and strives to achieve the goals defined by the patient and family. Often this requires that team members cross boundaries and remain flexible in their role.

    B. Incorrect: The roles of the team must be complementary to each other not independent of the other disciplines.

    C. **Correct**: The team members reflect unique expertise that is integrated into a coordinated team approach focused on the individualized plan of care to achieve the goals as defined by the patient and family.

    D. Incorrect: Although team members are charged with the responsibility to function within professional boundaries, emotional attachments do occur and are acceptable within those boundaries.

49. The chaplain or pastoral care person on the IDT is

    A. Expected to be open to a wide range of values and beliefs

    B. Always the bereavement coordinator

    C. Expected to promote his or her own tenets of faith

    D. Responsible for assuring a peaceful death

Disease Progression

50. The late symptomatic stage of HIV is characterized by a CD4 count of

    A. > 100,000

    B. < 500

    C. < 200

    D. < 50

51. Signs and symptoms of advanced cancer include asthenia, which is defined as

    A. Loss of appetite with increasing weight loss

    B. Loss of strength with increasing weakness and debility

    C. Generation of new blood vessels to supply a tumor

    D. Decreased sense of taste and smell

49. Answer is A

A. **Correct**: The chaplain or pastoral care person must be flexible and open minded to meet the spiritual needs of the patient and family. Often this responsibility extends beyond the individual beliefs of the pastoral care person.

B. Incorrect: The bereavement coordinator can be the chaplain, a counselor, a volunteer or any other team member responsible for this care.

C. Incorrect: None of the team members should promote their own tenets of faith. This extends beyond one's professional boundaries.

D. Incorrect: Although the chaplain or pastoral care person is responsible for the spiritual needs of the patient and family, it is the responsibility of the whole IDT to assure a peaceful death.

Disease Progression

50. Answer is C

A. Incorrect: >100,000 is a measure of viral load, not CD4 count in the progression of HIV/AIDS.

B. Incorrect: A CD4 <500 is the early symptomatic stage.

C. **Correct**: The CD4 count is less than 200 cells/mm3 and the viral load is >100,000/ml in late symptomatic stage.

D. Incorrect: In advanced HIV disease the count is less than 50.

51. Answer is B

A. Incorrect: Anorexia is defined by loss of appetite and weight loss.

B. **Correct**: Asthenia is defined as debility, loss of strength and weakness.

C. Incorrect: Angiogenesis is the generation of blood vessels around the primary tumor.

D. Incorrect: Loss of taste and smell may be a contributory factor in anorexia but not asthenia.

52. Chemotherapy is most often used in palliative cancer care to

    A. Decrease the tumor burden and eliminate metastases

    B. Improve survival and the possibility of remission

    C. Reduce nausea by decreasing cell division in the CTZ

    D. Enhance comfort and symptom control

53. Your patient presents to the clinic with signs and symptoms of hematuria, dull flank pain and tenderness, and weight loss. You anticipate that the diagnosis could be

    A. Renal cancer

    B. Colon polyps

    C. Leukemia

    D. Lymphoma

54. The most life threatening complication of end stage cancer is

    A. Spinal cord compression

    B. Intracerebral metastasis

    C. Arterial hemorrhage

    D. Superior vena cava syndrome

52.   Answer is D

      A. Incorrect: Curative care attempts to decrease tumor burden and eliminate metastases.

      B. Incorrect: Chemotherapy is used to control disease and improve survival earlier in the illness course.

      C. Incorrect: Chemotherapy may increase nausea through direct effects on the CTZ.

      D. **Correct**: The goal of palliative care is to improve quality of life by enhancing comfort and symptom control.

53.   Answer is A

      A. **Correct**: Signs and symptoms of advanced renal cancer include gross hematuria, dull aching pain, palpable abdominal mass, fever, weight loss, elevated ESR and/or anemia and dyspnea.

      B. Incorrect: Relevant signs and symptoms of colon polyps would be rectal bleeding and possible changes in elimination.

      C. Incorrect: Signs and symptoms of leukemia include signs of infection, anemia, and unexplained bleeding.

      D. Incorrect: Signs and symptoms of advanced lymphoma include lymphadenopathy and night sweats, fevers and/or weight loss.

54.   Answer is C

      A. Incorrect: Spinal cord compression can be life threatening, but the primary concern is paralysis.

      B. Incorrect: Some cerebral metastases can be treated with palliative radiation therapy.

      C. **Correct**: Arterial hemorrhage either internally or externally is often a terminal event if the hemorrhage is massive.

      D. Incorrect: SVC syndrome can be palliated with radiation therapy.

55.   Neurological symptoms from spinal cord compression or cerebral metastases may improve with

    A. Antihypertensives

    B. Steroids

    C. Fluids

    D. Aspirin

56.   Signs and symptoms of left sided heart failure include

    A. Weight gain, peripheral edema, weakness

    B. Dyspnea, chest pain, flushing

    C. Nocturia, distant heart sounds, anxiety

    D. Anxiety, orthopnea, cough

57.   End stage respiratory disease usually leads to

    A. Breathlessness and limited activity

    B. Exertional dyspnea and weight gain

    C. Tachycardia and bradypnea

    D. Increased sputum and robust cough

55. Answer is B

   A. Incorrect: There is no beneficial effect of antihypertensives on intracranial pressure.

   B. **Correct**: Steroids such as dexamethasone are often used in late stage neurological events to reduce edema and minimize extension of tissue damage.

   C. Incorrect: Fluids may be restricted, not given.

   D. Incorrect: Thromboembolic strokes may be prevented with regular use of aspirin but aspirin will not have an effect on decreasing intracranial pressure.

56. Answer is D

   A. Incorrect: Weakness or fatigue is a symptom of left sided heart failure but weight gain and peripheral edema are indicative of right sided heart failure.

   B. Incorrect: Dyspnea is a symptom of left sided heart failure but chest pain and flushing are not.

   C. Incorrect: Nocturia is a symptom of right sided heart failure.

   D. **Correct**: Anxiety, orthopnea and cough are all indicative of left sided heart failure along with restlessness, dyspnea, nocturnal dyspnea, hemoptysis, tachycardia, wheezes, fatigue, and cyanosis or pallor.

57. Answer is A

   A. **Correct**: Signs and symptoms of end stage respiratory disease include decreased PO_2, increased PCO_2, fatigue and limited tolerance for activity, profound breathlessness, poor quality of life, weight loss and tachycardia.

   B. Incorrect: Weight gain is not a sign of end stage respiratory disease.

   C. Incorrect: Both tachycardia and tachypnea are exhibited at end stage.

   D. Incorrect: A robust cough is not a sign of end stage disease.

58. Ascites is a common finding of which end stage disease?

    A. Renal

    B. Hepatic

    C. Respiratory

    D. Coronary

59. The cause of death in patients with general debility is

    A. Multi-organ failure

    B. Hemorrhage

    C. Immobility

    D. Diabetes

60. Mr. Hayes is admitted to your hospice program with a diagnosis of AIDS. As you review and prioritize his current medications, you note that ganciclovir should be continued if possible to prevent which condition?

    A. Pneumocystis carinii

    B. Progressive multifocal leukoencephalopathy (PML)

    C. Toxoplasmosis

    D. CMV retinitis

58.	Answer is B

A.	Incorrect: Ascites is not a finding in end stage renal disease.

B.	**Correct**: Ascites is a significant characteristic of end stage hepatic disease along with jaundice, fatigue and encephalopathy.

C.	Incorrect: Signs and symptoms of end stage respiratory disease include decreased PO_2, increased PCO_2, fatigue and limited tolerance for activity, profound breathlessness, poor quality of life, weight loss, and tachycardia.

D.	Incorrect: Signs and symptoms of advanced cardiac disease are primarily fatigue, dyspnea, palpitation, and anginal pain even at rest.

59.	Answer is A

A.	**Correct**: Patients with general debility exhibit signs and symptoms of multiple organ impairment and impending failure along with complications of immobility.

B.	Incorrect: Hemorrhage is a cause of death where tumor growth impinges on arterial blood vessels.

C.	Incorrect: Immobility leads to complications that may hasten death in debilitated patients but is not the cause of death.

D.	Incorrect: Diabetes is frequently a comorbid condition, which can contribute to poorer patient outcomes but is not a cause of death in debility.

60.	Answer is D

A.	Incorrect: PCP is usually treated with sulfa as a primary agent and pentamidine for secondary treatment.

B.	Incorrect: There is no effective treatment for PML and this viral infection causing neurologic deficits may be treated with investigational agents.

C.	Incorrect: Protozoal infections are usually treated with sulfa.

D.	**Correct**: A viral infection attacking the eyes, CMV is most commonly treated with ganciclovir.

61. Which of the following cancers is the **LEAST** likely to metastasize to the bone?

   A. Colon

   B. Lung

   C. Prostate

   D. Breast

62. Which of the following cancers is the **LEAST** likely to metastasize to the brain?

   A. Breast

   B. Prostate

   C. Lung

   D. Kidney

63. You are called to the home of a patient with lung cancer who has the following signs and symptoms: headache, facial edema, hoarseness, dyspnea, and edematous arms. What is most likely happening with this patient?

   A. Pleural effusion

   B. Cardiac tamponade

   C. Syndrome of inappropriate anti-diuretic hormone (SIADH)

   D. Superior vena cava syndrome

61. Answer is A

A. **Correct**: Colon cancer is the least likely to metastasize to bone.

B. Incorrect: Lung commonly metastasizes to bone.

C. Incorrect: Prostate commonly metastasizes to bone.

D. Incorrect: Breast commonly metastasizes to bone.

62. Answer is B

A. Incorrect: Breast cancer commonly metastasizes to brain.

B. **Correct**: Of this list, prostate is the LEAST likely to metastasize to the brain. Common sites of distant metastases can be predicted from the pattern of venous drainage in the region of the tumor.

C. Incorrect: Lung cancer commonly metastasizes to brain.

D. Incorrect: Kidney cancer can also metastasize to brain.

63. Answer is D

A. Incorrect: Pleural effusion is an accumulation of fluid in the pleural space surrounding the lung, which may result in dyspnea but would not result in the other signs/symptoms mentioned.

B. Incorrect: Cardiac tamponade is an accumulation of blood or fluid around the pericardium. Dyspnea and hoarseness are signs/symptoms and others include chest pain, cough, dysphagia, and muffled heart sounds.

C. Incorrect: Signs and symptoms of SIADH include weight gain, weakness, lethargy, irritability, and hyponatremia.

D. **Correct**: These are classic signs of SVCS, an oncologic emergency requiring immediate attention.

64.	A 53-year-old man with lung cancer complains of increased pain in his right hip, aggravated by movement and more noticeable at night. When he walks and stands, the pain is greater. He also indicates there is local tenderness on palpation. These are all signs/symptoms of probable

A.	Bone metastasis

B.	Impaired bone marrow function

C.	Hypercalcemia

D.	Paget's disease

65.	Which of the following infections is the most common in hospice patients?

A.	Septicemia

B.	Pneumonia

C.	Wound infection

D.	Influenza

66.	Which cell type is primarily affected by the AIDS virus

A.	B-lymphocytes

B.	Basophils

C.	Eosinophils

D.	T-lymphocytes

64.   Answer is A

   A. **Correct**: These are classic signs of bone metastasis.

   B. Incorrect: Bone marrow impairment manifests itself through altered hematology lab values—WBCs, RBCs and platelets.

   C. Incorrect: Hypercalcemia is commonly associated with lethargy, constipation, anorexia, confusion, and polyuria but not pain.

   D. Incorrect: Paget's disease is an inflammatory bone disease manifested by bone deterioration. Local tenderness would be an unusual symptom.

65.   Answer is B

   A. Incorrect: Although septicemia is a major life threatening infection, it is not the most common.

   B. **Correct**: Pneumonia is common among hospice patients, because the patient is debilitated and therefore less active, making them a high risk candidate.

   C. Incorrect: With good nursing and personal care and palliative treatment most patients can avoid wound infections.

   D. Incorrect: While debilitated patients may be susceptible to influenza, this is not the most common infection.

66.   Answer is D

   A. Incorrect: B-lymphocytes produce antigen-specific antibodies and are not affected by the AIDS virus.

   B. Incorrect: Basophils are a type of neutrophil not affected by the AIDS virus.

   C. Incorrect: Eosinophils are a type of neutrophil not affected by the AIDS virus.

   D. **Correct**: The virus has a high affinity for attaching to the CD4 cell surface protein of T-4 lymphocytes.

67. Which of the following infections is common in patients with AIDS unless treated prophylactically?

   A. Aspergillus

   B. MAI/MAC

   C. Salmonellosis

   D. Pneumocystis pneumonia

68. Of the following statements, which is the most accurate regarding AIDS dementia?

   A. Is a late occurring adverse effect of antiretroviral therapy

   B. May be completely reversed with antiretroviral treatment

   C. Is a poor prognostic sign and indicative of advanced disease

   D. Occurs in all patients with AIDS

69. Which of the following are the most common malignancies associated with HIV disease?

   A. CNS lymphoma, non-Hodgkin's lymphoma

   B. Colorectal cancer, Kaposi's sarcoma

   C. Multiple myeloma, leukemia

   D. Glioblastoma, melanoma

67.   Answer is D

   A. Incorrect: Pneumocystis pneumonia is developed by 85% of AIDS patients without proper treatment.

   B. Incorrect: Same as A

   C. Incorrect: Same as A

   D. **Correct**: Pneumocystis carinii pneumonia is a very common complication of AIDS and can be treated prophylactically.

68.   Answer is C

   A. Incorrect: AIDS dementia complex is a direct result of the disease, not the treatment for it.

   B. Incorrect: AIDS dementia is not reversible although retrovirals can delay onset.

   C. **Correct**: HIV directly damages the nervous tissue resulting in AIDS dementia and long term prognosis is poor.

   D. Incorrect: Not all AIDS patients develop AIDS dementia.

69.   Answer is A

   A. **Correct**: Both non-Hodgkin's lymphoma and CNS lymphoma have a higher incidence in patients with HIV disease.

   B. Incorrect: While Kaposi's sarcoma, a malignancy of soft/connective tissue marked by brownish purple popular lesions is common, colorectal cancer is not.

   C. Incorrect: Uncommonly seen in AIDS patients.

   D. Incorrect: The common brain tumor in HIV disease is CNS lymphoma, not glioblastoma.

70. Which three symptoms describe the early signs of spinal cord compression? Back pain and

   A. Paraplegia, urinary hesitancy

   B. Loss of rectal sensation, urinary retention

   C. Leg weakness, "funny feelings" in legs

   D. Decreased level of consciousness, paralysis

71. Which oncologic emergency is aggressively treated in hospice care?

   A. Tumor lysis syndrome

   B. Syndrome of inappropriate anti-diuretic hormone (SIADH)

   C. Hypercalcemia

   D. Spinal cord compression

72. The general effects of chemotherapy include bone marrow suppression, alopecia, and GI effects because

   A. Chemotherapy is circulated throughout the circulatory system

   B. Chemotherapeutic agents affect cells that are rapidly dividing

   C. Bone marrow suppression, alopecia, and GI effects occur as a result of the cancer itself, not the chemotherapy

   D. Chemotherapeutic agents kill cells in the bone marrow, hair follicles, stomach, and intestines because these are highly vascularized areas where metastatic cancer cells are in abundance

70. Answer is C

    A. Incorrect: Paraplegia is a late sign of cord compression.

    B. Incorrect: Loss of rectal sensation is a late sign of cord compression.

    C. **Correct**: These symptoms are classic for early signs of spinal cord compression and require immediate treatment to prevent paraplegia.

    D. Incorrect: Paralysis is a late sign of cord compression and the individual's level of consciousness is not affected at any time by the cord compression.

71. Answer is D

    A. Incorrect: Tumor Lysis Syndrome is an oncologic emergency secondary to chemotherapy and therefore would be highly unlikely in hospice care.

    B. Incorrect: SIADH may be treated to relieve symptoms but is not aggressively managed in hospice care.

    C. Incorrect: Hypercalcemia may be treated to relieve symptoms but is not aggressively managed in hospice care.

    D. **Correct**: Spinal cord compression can progress to paraplegia if not aggressively managed and therefore even in hospice care is considered an emergency that may require immediate intervention.

72. Answer is B

    A. Incorrect: Although this is true, it does not explain these specific effects.

    B. **Correct**: Bone marrow, hair and GI cells have rapid turnover due to the rapid mitotic rate and therefore are more specifically affected.

    C. Incorrect: These are side effects of chemotherapy not effects of the malignancy.

    D. Incorrect: These are all areas with rapidly dividing cells, not necessarily with high numbers of metastatic cells.

73. Hypercalcemia is commonly seen in late stages of which diseases?

    A. Breast cancer, multiple myeloma

    B. Pancreatic cancer, prostate cancer

    C. Colon cancer, ovarian cancer

    D. Leukemia, non-Hodgkin's lymphoma

74. Breast cancer commonly metastasizes to which sites?

    A. Pancreas, bone, brain

    B. Lymph nodes, pancreas, liver

    C. Lung, liver, bone

    D. Brain, bone, spleen

75. Advanced symptoms of end stage liver disease include

    A. Infection, pruritis, azotemia

    B. Jaundice, dyspnea, increased albumin levels

    C. Bleeding, nausea/vomiting, decreased bilirubin levels

    D. Fatigue, ascites, encephalopathy

73. Answer is A

    A. **Correct**: Hypercalcemia is caused by increased bone resorption due to osteoclast activity which is a) stimulated by the tumor, b) a direct result of invasion of the bone by tumor, c) decreased ability of the kidney to clear calcitonin and/or d) increased calcium absorption from the gut.

    B. Incorrect: Pancreatic cancer rarely affects the bones.

    C. Incorrect: Colon cancer rarely affects the bones.

    D. Incorrect: Leukemia rarely affects the bones.

74. Answer is C

    A. Incorrect: Breast cancer does not metastasize to pancreas.

    B. Incorrect: Breast cancer does not metastasize to pancreas.

    C. **Correct**: Lung, liver and bone are the common sites for metastasis of breast cancer.

    D. Incorrect: Breast cancer would not usually metastasize to the spleen.

75. Answer is D

    A. Incorrect: Azotemia is a sign of renal failure.

    B. Incorrect: Jaundice appears as the bile builds up in the blood but albumin levels decrease in end stage liver disease. Liver failure disables the function of protein catabolism.

    C. Incorrect: Bilirubin levels do not decrease.

    D. **Correct**: Fatigue is the hallmark symptom of chronic hepatitis. Ascites is the result of excess fluids, no longer draining through the lymphatics, leaking into the abdominal cavity. Encephalopathy is an early stage of hepatic coma.

76. Which side effect of chemotherapy can be asymptomatic but has serious life-threatening potential?

   A. Bone marrow suppression—especially the white cells, making the patient susceptible to infections

   B. Epithelial denudement of the gastrointestinal tract

   C. Bone marrow suppression—especially the red cells, making the patient susceptible to anemia

   D. Weight loss

Pain Management

77. Pain that is described as well localized with a deep, dull and achy quality is

   A. Visceral pain

   B. Somatic pain

   C. Neuropathic pain

   D. Nociceptive pain

78. Which of the following pain assessment parameters is most important to obtain as it directly correlates with the patient's quality of life?

   A. Location

   B. Duration

   C. Onset

   D. Intensity

76.   Answer is A

   A. **Correct**: Neutropenia is silent but dangerous leaving no neutrophils to fight the threat of infections. Neutropenia can be the cause of a septic situation, which is life threatening.

   B. Incorrect: Denudement of the GI tract is usually very symptomatic with mouth ulcers, heartburn, nausea, diarrhea.

   C. Incorrect: Anemia is concerning but not as immediately dangerous as neutropenia.

   D. Incorrect: Weight loss may occur without distress to the patient. In the long run, anorexia and cachexia can lead to debility and death but weight loss is not life-threatening in the short term.

Pain Management

77.   Answer is B

   A. Incorrect: Visceral pain is poorly localized and described as cramping, deep ache, and pressure.

   B. **Correct**: Somatic pain is well localized and often described as a deep, dull ache.

   C. Incorrect: Neuropathic pain is described as sharp, burning, shooting, and/or shock-like.

   D. Incorrect: Nociceptive pain is somatic and visceral pain.

78.   Answer is D

   A. Incorrect: Location, while important does not directly impact upon daily function and quality of life.

   B. Incorrect: Duration, while important does not directly impact upon daily function and quality of life.

   C. Incorrect: Onset, while important does not directly impact upon daily function and quality of life.

   D. **Correct**: As pain intensity increases, so does the negative impact on the patient's quality of life and daily function

79. How many patients with advanced disease experience pain?

    A. 30 to 50%

    B. 50 to 70%

    C. 70 to 90%

    D. 100%

80. Which of the following statements is true?

    A. Addiction to pain medications is common

    B. Adequately controlling symptoms at end of life does not shorten life

    C. The principle of double effect is applicable to end-of-life care

    D. Respiratory depression is a common adverse effect of opioids

81. Which of the following treatment modalities are appropriate for the primary treatment of severe, constant pain?

    A. Sustained-release opioids

    B. Nerve blocks

    C. Transcutaneous nerve stimulation

    D. Adjuvant analgesics

79.   Answer is C

   A. Incorrect: Answer is C

   B. Incorrect: Answer is C

   C. **Correct**: Pain is experienced by 70 to 90% of persons with advanced disease.

   D. Incorrect: Answer is C

80.   Answer is B

   A. Incorrect: Addiction is rare when opioids are used to treat pain.

   B. **Correct**: Research has demonstrated that adequately controlling symptoms at end of life does not shorten life or hasten death.

   C. Incorrect: The principle of double effect is often erroneously applied to end of life. Research has demonstrated that adequately controlling symptoms at end of life does not shorten life or hasten death.

   D. Incorrect: Respiratory depression is only a concern with persons who are opioid-naive. Tolerance to the respiratory depressant effect of opioids develops rapidly.

81.   Answer is A

   A. **Correct**: Opioids are the mainstay of the treatment of severe pain.

   B. Incorrect: While nerve blocks or other kinds of special procedures may be helpful in the treatment of severe pain, they are not considered primary, first-line therapy.

   C. Incorrect: Transcutaneous nerve stimulation is most appropriate for mild pain.

   D. Incorrect: While adjuvant analgesics should be considered as part of the regimen, they are not the mainstay treatment of severe pain.

82. Which of the following is the best description of addiction?

    A. The need for increasing doses of an opioid to maintain original analgesic effect

    B. A condition with genetic, psychologic, and environmental factors

    C. A syndrome where a patient makes frequent demands for opioids

    D. The onset of agitation, irritability, abdominal cramping, diarrhea, and piloerection

83. Which of the following agents is **NOT** anti-inflammatory?

    A. Dexamethasone

    B. Ibuprofen

    C. Acetaminophen

    D. Aspirin

84. Adverse effects of NSAIDs include

    A. Hepatotoxicity

    B. Diarrhea

    C. Respiratory depression

    D. Headache

82.   Answer is B

    A. Incorrect: This is tolerance. People with addictive disease using opioids to obtain euphoric effect experience tolerance.

    B. **Correct**: Addiction is a primary, chronic, neurobiologic disease with genetic, psychosocial, and environment factors influencing its development and manifestations.

    C. Incorrect: This is pseudoaddiction. Patients with pain appropriately request additional medication.

    D. Incorrect: These are signs and symptoms of the abstinence (or withdrawal) syndrome and occur when an individual rapidly discontinues the drug or an antagonist is given.

83.   Answer is C

    A. Incorrect: Dexamethasone is strongly anti-inflammatory.

    B. Incorrect: Ibuprofen is anti-inflammatory.

    C. **Correct**: Acetaminophen is analgesic and antipyretic but not anti-inflammatory.

    D. Incorrect: Aspirin is anti-inflammatory.

84.   Answer is D

    A. Incorrect: This is an adverse effect of high doses of acetaminophen, which is not an NSAID.

    B. Incorrect: NSAIDs cause gastrointestinal bleeding but do not necessarily increase or decrease frequency of bowel movements.

    C. Incorrect: NSAIDs have no known effect on respiration.

    D. **Correct**: NSAIDs can cause headaches, which may be due in part to changes in blood pressure due to decreased renal function.

85. Which of the following opioids is the most useful in hospice or palliative care?

A. Meperidine

B. Propoxyphene

C. Butorphanol tartrate

D. Methadone

86. The nurse is reviewing hospital discharge orders for a client who will begin hospice care at home. The client has terminal lung cancer and bone metastasis. He has been reluctant to move about because of pain. The client is receiving sustained release morphine 30 mg every 12 hours PO, but has an IV access device in case parenteral medication is needed. Which order should the nurse question?

A. Morphine 10 mg IV every 4 hours if client is vomiting

B. Ibuprofen 600 mg PO every 6 hours

C. Morphine 10 mg PO every 4 hours PRN for break through pain

D. Gabapentin 300 mg PO three times a day

87. A patient with chronic cancer pain has been receiving morphine 100 mg/hour intravenously for 2 months. Yesterday the dose was increased to 125 mg/hour to provide adequate pain control. Which of the following adverse effects is most likely to occur?

A. Respiratory depression

B. Constipation

C. Nausea

D. Itching

85. Answer is D

   A. Incorrect: Meperidine has poor oral bioavailability and neurotoxic metabolites (normeperidine) accumulate in renal dysfunction.

   B. Incorrect: Propoxyphene is a weak opioid, usually in admixtures with significant doses of acetaminophen (e.g., 650 mg) and the metabolite may produce tumors.

   C. Incorrect: Mixed agonist-antagonists have a ceiling dose, are associated with psychomimetic effects and may reverse the effect of any pure agonist opioids (e.g., morphine) previously given to the patient.

   D. **Correct**: Methadone is useful in pain control, safe with careful titration, and inexpensive.

86. Answer is A

   A. **Correct**: The nurse should question this order. This is an inappropriate equianalgesic dose for IV morphine for pain control.

   B. Incorrect: This is an appropriate dosage of ibuprofen and could be included in the pain regimen for treatment of metastatic bone pain.

   C. Incorrect: This is an appropriate breakthrough dosage of oral morphine (10-20% of 24 hour dose).

   D. Incorrect: This could be an appropriate adjuvant analgesic for the treatment of neuropathic pain in lung cancer, especially when the brachial plexus is involved.

87. Answer is B

   A. Incorrect: Since the patient has been on high dose morphine for chronic pain for a lengthy period respiratory depression is not a concern.

   B. **Correct**: Tolerance is not developed to the side effect of constipation and nurses must be vigilant in maintaining adequate elimination when a patient is on high doses of opioids.

   C. Incorrect: Tolerance to the side effect of nausea usually develops in long term use of opioids.

   D. Incorrect: Itching is not a common side effect.

88. Mr. F has advanced prostate cancer with bone metastasis. He is unresponsive and is being cared for at home by his daughter. The home health nurse is teaching the daughter about assessing her father's pain. Which statement by the daughter indicates understanding of her father's pain status?

   A. "If he is not moaning, he's probably not experiencing pain."

   B. "I'll have to guess when he is in pain since he can't tell me."

   C. "Now that he's unable to communicate, we can stop his pain medication."

   D. "Since he was in pain when he was conscious, I assume he's still in pain."

89. The nurse is conducting a pain assessment for a female client with liver cancer. The client is complaining of right shoulder pain that is rated as a 9 on a 0 to 10 pain scale. Which action should the nurse take first?

   A. Assess the patient's use of the prescribed pain medication

   B. Offer her a back massage to help her relax and decrease the pain

   C. Place hot packs to the right shoulder to reduce localized pain

   D. Perform an assessment of her pulse and respiratory rate

90. The nurse is talking with the parents of a 2-year-old boy diagnosed with leukemia about pain management. Which statement by the nurse indicates understanding about pain management in children?

   A. "He is at risk for addiction due to his early exposure to pain medications."

   B. "He may require less analgesia since he has limited memory of the pain."

   C. "He needs to be assessed carefully so that he gets enough pain medication."

   D. "He doesn't have full pain sensitivity due to an underdeveloped nervous system."

88. Answer is D

   A. Incorrect: In the setting of chronic pain patients may not exhibit typical behaviors associated with acute pain.

   B. Incorrect: The caregiver can assess pain by being alert to changes in behavior.

   C. Incorrect: If the patient has been in pain, continued pain should be assumed and treated.

   D. **Correct**: As the cause of his pain is still present, we can assume that he is still in pain.

89. Answer is A

   A. **Correct**: A patient in severe pain needs immediate analysis of the pharmacological management.

   B. Incorrect: Non-pharmacologic measures are not appropriate as a first action in the setting of severe pain.

   C. Incorrect: See B

   D. Incorrect: Vital signs are not relevant in the setting of chronic pain.

90. Answer is C

   A. Incorrect: Risk for addiction is not related to the age of the patient.

   B. Incorrect: Children experience pain and have memory of it.

   C. **Correct**: Lack of a careful assessment and underdosing can lead to pain that is out of control and difficult to manage.

   D. Incorrect: See B

91. The nurse is admitting a client with shingles. The client complains of a burning pain in the abdominal region that is rated a 7 on a 0 to 10 scale. The client had taken the prescribed opioid analgesic an hour ago just prior to admission. Which action should the nurse take?

    A. Administer medication prescribed for breakthrough pain

    B. Apply a warm compress to the affected abdominal region

    C. Gently massage the area surrounding the affected abdominal area

    D. Obtain a prescription for ibuprofen 400 mg PRN every four hours

92. The nurse is admitting a client with metastatic breast cancer. The client has bleeding gums and guaiac positive stools. The client has an elevated temperature and a respiratory rate of 10 per minute. The client is complaining of aching and throbbing pain in the right femur. Which order should the nurse question?

    A. Administer morphine 60 mg PO every 4 hours for 24 hours

    B. Institute bleeding precautions

    C. Apply a transdermal fentanyl patch 25 mcg/per hour every 72 hours

    D. Give ibuprofen 400 mg every 4 hours for an elevated temperature

93. Which statement by the nurse indicates a correct understanding of pain management for clients with a history of substance abuse?

    A. "They should not be given opioids for pain because of the high addiction risk."

    B. "They will need smaller doses of analgesia to prevent cumulative overdose."

    C. "They may require higher does of opioids to relieve their pain."

    D. "They need to withdraw from the substance prior to receiving analgesia."

91.	Answer is A

    A.	**Correct**: The patient should have orders for an analgesic to be given on a PRN basis for break-through pain. This would be the first action of the nurse.

    B.	Incorrect: This is not an effective therapy for immediate relief of neuropathic pain.

    C.	Incorrect: See B

    D.	Incorrect: Ibuprofen is not indicated as an adjuvant analgesic for neuropathic pain.

92.	Answer is D

    A.	Incorrect: This would be an appropriate order for immediate release morphine for breakthrough pain.

    B.	Incorrect: This would be appropriate given the findings of bleeding gums and guaiac positive stools.

    C.	Incorrect: This would be an appropriate order for management of chronic pain.

    D.	**Correct**: This would be questioned because of the patient's risk for bleeding.

93.	Answer is C

    A.	Incorrect: Patients with a history of substance abuse still have a right to pain relief.

    B.	Incorrect: There is no cumulative overdose; there is no ceiling dose for opioids.

    C.	**Correct**: Tolerance to medications may be higher in persons with previous exposure.

    D.	Incorrect: See A

94. The nurse is caring for Ms. P, a 55-year-old woman with cancer. She received pain medication less than two hours ago after which she expressed significant relief. A colleague now reports that Mrs. P is complaining of pain. The colleague says "She can't be hurting as much as she says she is." What is the nurse's most appropriate response?

   A. "We need to explore the cultural meaning pain has for her."

   B. "Pain is whatever she says it is. Let's assess her further."

   C. "I will tell her gently that she must wait four hours between doses."

   D. "I'll wait to give the next dose and re-assess her a little early, in an hour."

95. Objective or observational assessment of pain or discomfort in the non-responsive patient includes what indicators?

   A. Behavioral

   B. Psychological

   C. Previous subjective assessment including physical signs and symptoms

   D. All of the above

96. What is the maximum recommended dose of acetaminophen per day?

   A. 4 Grams

   B. 6 Grams

   C. 1000 mg

   D. 650 mg

94. Answer is B

   A. Incorrect: This response is not related to the colleague's statement.

   B. **Correct**: The patient's report of pain is the starting point for pain assessment and management.

   C. Incorrect: The nurse must take action to achieve an acceptable level of pain relief for the patient.

   D. Incorrect: See C

95. Answer is D

   A. Incorrect: Must include all three: behavioral, psychological, and previous subjective assessment.

   B. Incorrect: Assessment should include all previous subjective assessments as well as behavioral indicators.

   C. Incorrect: Behavioral and psychological indicators should also be considered including signs and symptoms.

   D. **Correct**: Behavioral, psychological and all previous subjective assessment information is most helpful in the non-responsive patient to properly assess the current discomforts.

96. Answer is A

   A. **Correct**: This is the maximum daily-recommended dose of acetaminophen. Many combination pain medications contain acetaminophen and should be considered in calculating the total daily dose.

   B. Incorrect: This equals 1.5 times of the maximum daily allowance.

   C. Incorrect: This equals one-fourth of the maximum daily allowance.

   D. Incorrect: This equals one-sixth the maximum daily allowance.

97.　When assessing a patient with neuropathic pain, verbal indicators may include the following descriptors

A. Shooting

B. Aching

C. Dull

D. Localized

98.　What types of pain typically require adjuvant analgesics?

A. Visceral

B. Somatic

C. Neuropathic

D. Nociceptive

99.　Mrs. A. is new to your hospice program. She has a diagnosis of metastatic breast cancer. She reports severe pain (9 on a 10 point scale) in her back and right upper quadrant area. The first thing you should do is

A. Start liquid morphine

B. Start morphine, sustained release

C. Call the doctor

D. Examine the patient and obtain a history

97.   Answer is A

   A. **Correct**: Shooting pain is the typical descriptor. Others may include sharp, tingling, electrical, burning.

   B. Incorrect: Somatic pain is aching, throbbing pain from bone, soft tissue, or internal organs.

   C. Incorrect: Chronic dull pain is not related to neuropathic pain.

   D. Incorrect: Localized describes the location rather than the type of pain.

98.   Answer is C

   A. Incorrect: Visceral pain requires opioids. It is squeezing, cramping pain of internal organs, soft tissues or bone.

   B. Incorrect: Somatic pain is aching, throbbing pain experienced in organs, soft tissues or bones, and benefits from opioids.

   C. **Correct**: Neuropathic pain is generally due to damage to the nervous system. Adjuvants are used to enhance the analgesic efficacy of opioids especially in cases of neuropathic pain. Antidepressants, anticonvulsants, and corticosteroids are examples of adjuvants.

   D. Incorrect: As indicated in the explanation for A and B since nociceptive pain includes both visceral and somatic.

99.   Answer is D

   A. Incorrect: Liquid morphine is immediate release and can be used for relief of pain but a thorough assessment must be performed first.

   B. Incorrect: Sustained release morphine is a long acting agent that requires multiple doses to establish serum steady state. Severe pain must have immediate release morphine.

   C. Incorrect: The assessment must be completed first before calling the physician for appropriate orders.

   D. **Correct**: The patient needs to be quickly assessed with a review of her history prior to calling the physician for the appropriate medication order.

100. When are non-pharmacologic interventions appropriate to use for pain control?

A. In place of opioids, when the patient is fearful of addiction

B. To augment optimal pharmacologic management

C. To give the family concrete tasks to care for the patient

D. To manage breakthrough pain

101. What are beneficial effects of NSAIDs in addition to anti-inflammatory properties?

A. Analgesic, antipyretic

B. Analgesic, serotonin inhibition

C. Analgesic, antispasmodic

D. Serotonin inhibition, antipyretic

102. What type of pain would benefit most from nortriptyline?

A. Smooth muscle spasms

B. Visceral

C. Neuropathic

D. Somatic

100.　Answer is B

    A.　Incorrect: The pharmacologic interventions are not replaced by non-pharmacologic interventions.

    B.　**Correct**: Yes, the non-pharmacologic interventions will augment the optimal pharmacologic management.

    C.　Incorrect: Pain relief requires pharmacologic interventions; family needs to be educated to understand pain management.

    D.　Incorrect: Non-pharmacologic interventions are not adequate for breakthrough pain.

101.　Answer is A

    A.　**Correct**: NSAIDs have anti-inflammatory, analgesic and antipyretic benefits.

    B.　Incorrect: NSAIDs do not inhibit serotonin.

    C.　Incorrect: NSAIDs are not antispasmodics.

    D.　Incorrect: NSAIDs do not inhibit serotonin.

102.　Answer is C

    A.　Incorrect: Nortriptyline will not benefit muscle spasms.

    B.　Incorrect: Visceral pain will not be relieved by nortriptyline.

    C.　**Correct**: Nortriptyline prevents the reuptake of serotonin and norepinephrine thereby inhibiting the transmission of the pain impulse. Side effects include drowsiness, dry mouth, urinary retention, and orthostatic hypotension.

    D.　Incorrect: Somatic pain will not be relieved by nortriptyline.

103. "If the gut works, use it" is frequently stated. When pain medications are given via the GI tract, what percentage of patients would obtain pain relief?

    A. 25%

    B. 50%

    C. 70%

    D. 90%

104. Which of the following drugs is **NOT** recommended for use in the management of chronic pain?

    A. Morphine

    B. Hydromorphone

    C. Meperidine

    D. Fentanyl

105. What is the ceiling dose of morphine?

    A. There is no ceiling dose of morphine

    B. 300 milligrams every 4 hours

    C. 600 milligrams every 4 hours

    D. 1000 milligrams every 4 hours

106. The state of adaptation in which exposure to a drug induces changes that result in a diminution of one or more of the drug's effects over time is the definition for

    A. Addiction

    B. Tolerance

    C. Physical dependence

    D. Pseudoaddiction

103. Answer is D

   A. Incorrect: More than 90% of individuals would obtain relief when medications are administered orally.

   B. Incorrect: See A

   C. Incorrect: See A

   D. **Correct**: If the gut works, use it! More than 90% of individuals with pain would benefit from oral pain medication.

104. Answer is C

   A. Incorrect: Morphine is the "gold standard" for chronic cancer pain.

   B. Incorrect: Hydromorphone is very effective with chronic pain.

   C. **Correct**: Normeperidine is the toxic metabolite of meperidine. Because normeperidine toxicity often appears after several days of treatment, this drug is not recommended for chronic use.

   D. Incorrect: Fentanyl is very effective in specific cases of chronic pain.

105. Answer is A

   A. **Correct**: Morphine has no ceiling dose. The dose gradually increases due to tolerance and/or disease progression.

   B. Incorrect: Morphine has no ceiling dose.

   C. Incorrect: Morphine has no ceiling dose.

   D. Incorrect: Morphine has no ceiling dose.

106. Answer is B

   A. Incorrect: Addiction is a primary, chronic, neurobiologic disease, with genetic, psychosocial, and environmental factors influencing its development and manifestations.

   B. **Correct**: This is the definition of tolerance.

   C. Incorrect: Physical dependence is a state of adaptation that is manifested by a drug class specific withdrawal syndrome that can be produced by abrupt cessation, rapid dose reduction, decreasing blood level of the drug, and/or administration of an antagonist.

   D. Incorrect: Pseudoaddiction is a result of undertreatment of pain causing the individual to appear to be a "drug seeker." In such cases, patients who have suffered prolonged, unrelieved pain may become more aggressive in seeking relief.

107. The dose limiting side effect of morphine in the patient receiving high doses for chronic pain is

    A. Respiratory depression

    B. Myoclonus

    C. Constipation

    D. Hallucinations

108. A cancer patient has been upwardly titrated on morphine within a short period of time without success in meeting pain relief goals. What is the most appropriate next step?

    A. Add an adjuvant analgesic

    B. Schedule for a nerve block

    C. Initiate sedation protocol for intractable pain

    D. Reassess patient for etiology of increased pain

109. A cancer patient has continued side effects from opioid therapy for bone pain that leads to a decreased quality of life and non-compliance with the pain regimen. What is another therapeutic option for this patient?

    A. NSAIDs/Cox-2 inhibitors

    B. Anticonvulsants

    C. Anesthetics

    D. Antidepressants

107. Answer is B

    A. Incorrect: Respiratory depression is a side effect, however, it is not dose limiting in the setting of chronic pain management.

    B. **Correct**: Opioids given in high doses may result in myoclonus as a result of elevated levels of morphine-3-glucuronide and morphine 6-glucuronide, which are neuroexcitatory metabolites of morphine.

    C. Incorrect: Constipation is experienced in all patients receiving opioids, but is very treatable.

    D. Incorrect: Hallucinations are more common when morphine is initiated.

108. Answer is D

    A. Incorrect: Another medication should not be started until a reassessment is completed.

    B. Incorrect: There is not enough information given to suggest that this would be an appropriate intervention without further assessment.

    C. Incorrect: Sedation is considered after all other options have been exhausted. The patient may benefit from a change to another opioid analgesic or the addition of other medications after further assessment.

    D. **Correct**: Reassessment is critical to developing the best plan for the patient and achieving success with pain relief.

109. Answer is A

    A. **Correct**: Bone pain responds well to anti-inflammatories and like medications.

    B. Incorrect: Anticonvulsants are appropriate in the management of neuropathic pain.

    C. Incorrect: See B

    D. Incorrect: See B

110. The responsibility for pain assessment and management lies with the

    A. Physician

    B. Nurse

    C. Family caregiver

    D. All team members

111. Which of the following is most likely to indicate pain in a nonverbal patient in the final days of life?

    A. Furrowed brow

    B. Irregular respirations

    C. Diaphoresis

    D. Moaning

Symptom Management

112. A pressure ulcer that involves the full thickness of skin is classified as a

    A. Stage I

    B. Stage II

    C. Stage III

    D. Stage IV

110. Answer is D

   A. Incorrect: While the physician has an important role in the assessment and management of pain, this is not the best answer.

   B. Incorrect: While the nurse has an important role in the assessment and management of pain, this is not the best answer.

   C. Incorrect: While the family caregiver has a unique role in the daily assessment and administration of medication, this is not the best answer.

   D. **Correct**: Responsibility for relieving pain is shared by all disciplines and the patient and family together as a team.

111. Answer is A

   A. **Correct**: A furrowed brow may be indicative of pain in the nonverbal patient.

   B. Incorrect: Irregular respirations would be expected at the end of life but would not necessarily indicate pain.

   C. Incorrect: Diaphoresis is not an indicator of pain.

   D. Incorrect: Regular or rhythmic moaning could be associated with pain but may like irregular respirations be a manifestation of imminent death.

Symptom Management

112. Answer is C

   A. Incorrect: A Stage I pressure ulcer is non-blanchable erythema of intact skin.

   B. Incorrect: A Stage II pressure ulcer is the loss of partial thickness of skin involving the epidermis, dermis or both.

   C. **Correct**: A Stage III pressure ulcer involves the full thickness of skin or necrosis of subcutaneous tissue that may extend down to but not through the fascia.

   D. Incorrect: A Stage IV pressure ulcer involved full thickness skin loss with extensive destruction, tissue necrosis or damage to muscle bone or supporting structures.

113. Which of the following can be used to decrease pruritus?

    A. Alcohol rubs

    B. Hot water

    C. Starch baths

    D. Thick clothing

114. Which is the best dressing for a wound that has only a small amount of exudate?

    A. Alginate

    B. Enzymatic

    C. Semipermeable film

    D. Hydrocolloid

115. According to his family, a 76-year-old man has become very confused "over night" and has been refusing to eat or drink for the past several days. Which of the following of his known medical conditions should be assessed first as a possible cause of his confusion?

    A. Benign prostatic hypertrophy

    B. Congestive heart failure

    C. History of alcoholism

    D. Irritable bowel syndrome

113. Answer is C

    A. Incorrect: Alcohol used topically can increase pruritus.

    B. Incorrect: Hot water can increase pruritus.

    C. **Correct**: Cool starch baths can decrease pruritus.

    D. Incorrect: Tight or heavy clothing can increase pruritus.

114. Answer is D

    A. Incorrect: An alginate dressing is best for wounds with heavy exudate to control secretions and bacterial contamination.

    B. Incorrect: An enzymatic dressing aids in loosening necrotic tissue by liquefaction.

    C. Incorrect: A semipermeable film is not absorbent and should not be used when there is exudate present. It can help protect early damage and assist with healing.

    D. **Correct**: A hydrocolloid would not work well on a wound with a large amount of exudate, but will fluidize into a gel that can assist with debridement and keep the wound bed moist to assist with granulation.

115. Answer is A

    A. **Correct**: Benign prostatic hypertrophy can cause urinary retention, which would lead to confusion in the elderly.

    B. Incorrect: Congestive heart failure may be a cause of his confusion, but he should be checked for a full bladder first.

    C. Incorrect: A history of alcoholism could provide an etiology for confusion/dementia, but not usually if it is sudden onset.

    D. Incorrect: Irritable bowel syndrome is most likely to cause diarrhea or loose stools. Constipation is a possible cause of confusion.

116. Corticosteroids are an effective appetite stimulant

    A. For short term use

    B. If nausea is not present

    C. Only in the terminal stages

    D. When early satiety is a problem

117. When teaching the family of a patient with ascites, which dietary modifications should be included?

    A. Increased fiber in the diet

    B. High protein diet

    C. Low protein diet

    D. Fluid and sodium restriction

118. Which of the following interventions would be effective for a patient with expressive aphasia from a cerebrovascular accident?

    A. Exercises taught by the speech pathologist

    B. Picture board

    C. Slow simple instructions

    D. Utilize eye blinking for yes or no

116. Answer is A

    A. **Correct**: Corticosteroids may lose effectiveness after a few weeks.

    B. Incorrect: Corticosteroids are useful in decreasing nausea and vomiting.

    C. Incorrect: Corticosteroids can be useful in all stages, but are not usually indicated in the terminal stages.

    D. Incorrect: Gastrokinetic agents would be more useful when early satiety is a problem.

117. Answer is D

    A. Incorrect: A high fiber diet may assist in preventing constipation but will not directly affect the accumulation of fluid.

    B. Incorrect: Though a decrease in plasma albumin may contribute to ascites, increasing protein in the diet will not reverse this process.

    C. Incorrect: Differences in dietary intake of protein will not affect the accumulation of fluid.

    D. **Correct**: A fluid and sodium restrictions may reduce the ascites.

118. Answer is B

    A. Incorrect: Exercises taught by the speech pathologist would be helpful with dysarthria.

    B. **Correct**: With expressive aphasia the patient understands what is being said and knows what they want to say, but is unable or limited in their ability to speak.

    C. Incorrect: The person with expressive aphasia understands what is being said.

    D. Incorrect: Eye blinking is useful in locked-in conditions where the patient maintains comprehension but has extremely limited neuromuscular function.

119. A 47-year-old with end stage bowel cancer has complaints of a "low abdominal cramping pain that has gotten worse since last night." This patient should be assessed for

A. Bowel strangulation

B. Ileus

C. Large bowel obstruction

D. Small bowel obstruction

120. Which of the following foods is recommended for a patient with diarrhea?

A. Applesauce

B. Coffee

C. Milkshakes

D. Whole grain breads

121. Which of the following is recommended to treat painful swallowing that is the result of esophagitis from radiotherapy?

A. Dexamethasone

B. Lidocaine/diphenhydrAMINE/antacid combination

C. Metoclopramide

D. Nystatin

119. Answer is C

    A. Incorrect: Severe, steady pain rather than cramping is more indicative of strangulation.

    B. Incorrect: An ileus is a cessation of peristalsis and is usually painless.

    C. **Correct**: A large bowel obstruction usually causes cramping pains in the lower abdomen that increase over time.

    D. Incorrect: Symptoms of a small bowel obstruction are cramping, colicky pains in the middle to upper abdomen relieved with vomiting.

120. Answer is A

    A. **Correct**: Applesauce is recommended to help keep the stool firm in consistency.

    B. Incorrect: Foods high in caffeine can increase the amount of water secreted by the intestines, thereby worsening the diarrhea.

    C. Incorrect: Milk contains lactulose, which can make the diarrhea worse.

    D. Incorrect: High-fiber foods should be avoided as they can decrease transit time in the large intestine.

121. Answer is B

    A. Incorrect: Steroids can be used to decrease inflammatory edema caused by tumors or nodes.

    B. **Correct**: A 1:1:1 ratio of lidocaine, diphenhydrAMINE and an antacid can decrease esophagitis from radiotherapy IF the patient has a gag reflex.

    C. Incorrect: Prokinetic agents may be used to treat poor esophageal motility.

    D. Incorrect: Antifungals may be used to treat candidiasis.

122. Which of the following should be included when teaching the patient about inhaled triamcinolone?

   A. Appetite will increase

   B. Avoid milk products

   C. Rinse and spit after each dose

   D. Stop if shortness of breath worsens

123. Myoclonus is best treated

   A. By opioid rotation

   B. Starting low dose diazepam

   C. Stopping adjuvant medications

   D. With gentle physical therapy

124. The drug of choice to relieve the patient's feeling of "air hunger" in end-stage pulmonary disease is

   A. Meperidine

   B. Lorazepam

   C. Dexamethasone

   D. Morphine

122. Answer is C

    A. Incorrect: Though triamcinolone is a steroid, it is only minimally absorbed systemically and should not have an effect on appetite.

    B. Incorrect: Milk products will have no effect on triamcinolone.

    C. **Correct**: Triamcinolone can cause thrush if left in the mouth. Rinsing and spitting after each dose will rinse the medications out of the mouth and decrease the risk of dysphonia.

    D. Incorrect: Any steroid should never be stopped suddenly. If shortness of breath worsens, contact the physician or call the hospice nurse.

123. Answer is A

    A. **Correct**: Myoclonus is induced by opioids. Changing the opioid can reduce the myoclonus.

    B. Incorrect: Diazepam will not have an effect on myoclonus.

    C. Incorrect: Adding adjuvant medications may reduce the amount of opioids needed to control pain.

    D. Incorrect: Physical therapy will not decrease or stop myoclonus.

124. Answer is D

    A. Incorrect: Meperidine should not be used in end stage diseases. Normeperidine is a toxic metabolite of meperidine that can build up with chronic administration and should be avoided.

    B. Incorrect: Lorazepam is indicated for anxiety, which can be useful where anxiety is a component of the patient's pattern of dyspnea. Although it could be helpful, it is not the best first medication to consider.

    C. Incorrect: While a steroid may be useful in treating asthma and COPD, it is not the best immediate first step to treat air hunger.

    D. **Correct**: Opioids provide palliative support for symptoms of breathlessness or suffocation even though the mechanism of action in dyspnea is not well understood.

125. Mrs. Jones has advanced lung cancer and is experiencing new shortness of breath. She has a past medical history of congestive heart failure and has been taking digoxin and furosemide. What is your first action in addressing her shortness of breath?

   A. Call the physician to request an order for morphine

   B. Call the physician to request an order for pulse oximmetry

   C. Inquire if the patient has been taking her medications for CHF

   D. Reassure the patient and family that this is part of the normal disease progression

126. Mrs. Smith is 54 years old and has end stage ovarian cancer. On your home visit today, she reports a 3-day history of vomiting. She has an increased abdominal girth and abdominal discomfort. Which of the following is the most likely cause?

   A. Gastroparesis

   B. Bowel obstruction

   C. Ileus

   D. Ascites

127. In reference to the previous question, to provide comfort for Mrs. Smith, all of the following choices are appropriate interventions **EXCEPT**

   A. NG tube to gravity

   B. Corticosteroids

   C. Metoclopramide

   D. Octreotide

125. Answer is C

    A. Incorrect: This is not appropriate until an assessment has been completed and possible etiologies examined.

    B. Incorrect: Same as A

    C. **Correct**: First conduct a complete assessment, which includes the patient's current physical exam findings, recent history, and compliance with the medication regimen.

    D. Incorrect: Until other treatable etiologies are ruled out, this would not be an appropriate action.

126. Answer is B

    A. Incorrect: Gastroparesis results in decreased intestinal motility but does not usually cause vomiting or abdominal discomfort.

    B. **Correct**: The classic symptoms of bowel obstruction are constipation, distension, abdominal discomfort, and vomiting.

    C. Incorrect: Ileus is usually painless.

    D. Incorrect: Anorexia and early satiety may be associated with ascites but not vomiting.

127. Answer is C

    A. Incorrect: An NG tube would prevent vomiting and therefore provide comfort but other measures are usually tried first.

    B. Incorrect: Corticosteroids can relieve obstruction especially if caused by metastatic disease progression.

    C. **Correct**: Metoclopramide would have no value since this patient has an obstruction and increased peristalsis could increase symptoms above the obstruction and would not alleviate the obstruction.

    D. Incorrect: Octreotide can actually reverse symptoms of small bowel obstruction.

128. Which of the following is helpful in the management of agitation?

    A. Provide stimulating music to divert the person's behavior

    B. Speak directly and distinctively into the person's ear to assure they hear you

    C. Postpone explanations for actions and interventions until the person is calm

    D. Maintain a calm, familiar environment with minimal stimuli

129. Skin that is blistered, cracked or abraded is what stage of skin breakdown?

    A. Stage I

    B. Stage II

    C. Stage III

    D. Stage IV

130. What is the appropriate skin care intervention for the skin breakdown described above?

    A. Surgical repair

    B. Irrigation and debridement

    C. Apply protective dressing

    D. Silvadene cream

131. Mr. Wilson has dysphagia subsequent to high-dose radiation therapy to the neck area. Which of the following is the most appropriate for his treatment plan?

    A. Liquids are always better tolerated in these patients

    B. Artificial saliva can be used ad lib for dysphagia

    C. The side effects of radiation therapy will resolve rapidly

    D. For mouth dryness, keep moistened with lemon and glycerin swabs

128.   Answer is D

   A. Incorrect: Music should be offered in soft calming tones.

   B. Incorrect: Spoken words should be offered in gentle tones to the person.

   C. Incorrect: You should explain all actions to the person.

   D. **Correct**: Maintaining a calm, familiar environment with minimal stimuli is the best non-prescriptive management of agitation.

129.   Answer is B

   A. Incorrect: Stage I is when the skin is deep pink, red, or mottled.

   B. **Correct**: Stage II is when the skin is blistered, cracked, or abraded.

   C. Incorrect: Stage III is when there is a crater like wound with involvement of the underlying tissues.

   D. Incorrect: Stage IV is when deep ulceration, necrosis, or wet/dry black exudates is present.

130.   Answer is C

   A. Incorrect: Surgical repair would be used on Stage IV wounds only.

   B. Incorrect: Irrigation and debridement is the therapy for Stage III wounds.

   C. **Correct**: The therapy for Stage II wounds is to relieve pressure and apply protective dressings.

   D. Incorrect: Silvadene would not be indicated in this situation.

131.   Answer is B

   A. Incorrect: The patient should be permitted to eat whatever he/she can tolerate.

   B. **Correct**: Dysphagia is difficulty swallowing. The artificial saliva will make swallowing easier.

   C. Incorrect: Side effects resolve slowly.

   D. Incorrect: Lemon adds to the mouth dryness and can be painful if there are inflamed areas secondary to radiation. Glycerin has an alcohol base and ultimately worsens dryness.

132. A hospice patient has been on corticosteroids for prolonged periods and exhibits night sweats, weight loss, and malaise. He may be exhibiting signs and symptoms of

   A. Tuberculosis

   B. Hepatitis B

   C. Human Immunodeficiency Virus (HIV)

   D. Lymphoma

133. A hospice nurse visits Mr. Tuttle, a 70-year-old man with CHF and cancer of the mouth. He is taking multiple drugs, including diuretics, anticholinergics, opioids, tranquilizers, antidepressants, and antihistamines. These could cause

   A. Stomatitis

   B. Xerostomia

   C. Dysphagia

   D. Esophagitis

134. Hypoxia manifests itself when the oxygen saturation drops to

   A. 95%

   B. 90%

   C. 85%

   D. Below 80%

135. Symptom management for dyspnea includes all of the following **EXCEPT**

   A. Keep room cool and control humidity

   B. Move air in room by fan or open window

   C. Encourage relaxation by gentle voice, gentle touching, and guiding slow deep breaths

   D. Position the patient in side-lying position with the bed flat

132. Answer is A

    A. **Correct**: These symptoms are classic for tuberculosis. Immunocompromised patients are at high risk for development of tuberculosis.

    B. Incorrect: Hepatitis B is a blood borne disease and is not usually associated with night sweats.

    C. Incorrect: HIV is a viral syndrome transmitted via blood from the infected person. HIV in the early stages has few or no symptoms associated with it.

    D. Incorrect: While these symptoms are associated with lymphoma, this is not the best answer given the situation.

133. Answer is B

    A. Incorrect: Stomatitis is inflammation of the oral cavity and is not usually caused by these medications.

    B. **Correct**: Xerostomia is dry mouth and can be caused by the interactions of multiple drugs that include antihistamines and anticholinergics.

    C. Incorrect: Dysphagia is difficulty swallowing not usually associated as a side effect of these medications.

    D. Incorrect: Esophagitis is inflammation of the esophageal lining and is not usually associated with these medications.

134. Answer is D

    A. Incorrect: Must be below 80%.

    B. Incorrect: Must be below 80%.

    C. Incorrect: Must be below 80%.

    D. **Correct**: Symptoms of hypoxia usually appear at this level. Patient's family members must be educated to understand the symptoms that may occur at this time.

135. Answer is D

    A. Incorrect: Keeping the room cool with control humidity is very helpful.

    B. Incorrect: Moving the air in the room is very comforting.

    C. Incorrect: Calm, relaxed atmosphere will assist with symptom management.

    D. **Correct**: Dyspnea is relieved by high Fowler's position and some patients will do better leaning forward with their arms supported on a table.

136. When should laxatives be initiated?

 A. After the patient has not experienced a bowel movement for five days

 B. When an enema is ineffective

 C. Upon initiation of an opioid

 D. When high fiber, fruits and bulk foods have failed

137. Mrs. L is admitted with end stage cancer and one of her problems is syncope. Which of the following should be done?

 A. Consider discontinuing antihypertensive medications if blood pressure is consistently low

 B. Encourage her to remain in bed

 C. Encourage her to drink less fluid to avoid needing to go to the bathroom

 D. Order a hospital bed with side rails and instruct family to keep them up at all times she is in bed

138. Which of the following statements about dyspnea at the end of life is **NOT** true?

 A. Occurs in the majority of advanced cancer patients

 B. May be relieved by a cool fan blowing on the patient

 C. Responds well to oxygen even in non-hypoxemic patients

 D. Is assessed primarily by the patient's description

136. Answer is C

    A. Incorrect: The patient's pattern of bowel movements should be maintained. Opioids decrease intestinal motility.

    B. Incorrect: If effective laxative agents are incorporated upon onset of opioid therapy, enemas should not be necessary.

    C. **Correct**: Opioids decrease intestinal motility therefore laxatives should be initiated when opioid therapy begins.

    D. Incorrect: Although these efforts promote normal elimination they are insufficient to overcome decreased intestinal motility associated with opioid administration.

137. Answer is A

    A. **Correct**: With end stage disease, blood pressure naturally decreases eliminating the need for continuing the antihypertensive medications. Syncope is usually related to orthostatic hypotension. Repeated blood pressure readings taken in the lying, sitting, standing positions would provide sufficient information to make a determination whether the antihypertensive medications could be decreased or discontinued.

    B. Incorrect: Although safety is a concern with this patient, we should not encourage her to remain in bed. Education of patient and family should include accompanying the patient when she is ambulating.

    C. Incorrect: Fluids are very important to prevent syncopal reactions. Dehydration is a common cause of orthostatic hypotension.

    D. Incorrect: Guardrails could possibly increase the risk of injury if the patient tries to climb over them. While guardrails may be appropriate once the patient is bed bound, the patient should be able to be as active as possible until the very end of life.

138. Answer is C

    A. Incorrect: Dyspnea does occur in the majority of advanced cancer patients.

    B. Incorrect: Dyspnea can be relieved by air movement.

    C. **Correct**: Oxygen may be given a therapeutic trial even in non-hypoxemic patients to see if there will be a benefit, but it is not generally effective.

    D. Incorrect: Dyspnea is the sensation of breathlessness and is best assessed by determining the patient's experience of it.

139. The nurse has admitted a client with ovarian cancer who has a pathologic hip fracture. The physician has increased the dosages of transdermal fentanyl and amitriptyline. It would be essential for the nurse to

A. Assess for pain relief and provide breakthrough medications

B. Assess the client for postural hypotension

C. Check the client's respirations hourly

D. Encourage the client to cough and deep breathe

140. Palliative nutrition means providing

A. Whatever the patient desires for comfort

B. Sufficient protein, calories and fat to regain optimal nutrition

C. A low-sodium diet to prevent edema

D. Enteral feedings when the patient is unable to swallow

141. The nurse has been assigned to care for a woman who was recently admitted for advanced cancer and who reports ongoing fatigue. Her husband offers observations about his wife's fatigue. Which statement by the husband indicates the most correct understanding of his wife's fatigue?

A. "She sleeps quite a bit, so she shouldn't be as tired as she is."

B. "She's lost some weight. I know she'll feel better if she eats more."

C. "She's been in pain. If we control that maybe she'll have more energy."

D. "She seems moody, so we need to cheer her up and make her laugh."

139. Answer is A

   A. **Correct**: The patient is receiving two long acting medications, an opioid and an adjuvant analgesic to manage pain. Reassessment is important to determine whether relief is obtained. The patient may experience pain with activity or movement and should have a PRN medication prescribed for break-through pain.

   B. Incorrect: Orthostatic hypotension can be a side effect of amitriptyline and the nurse should be aware of this, however, this is not the essential thing the nurse should be concerned with.

   C. Incorrect: The client is being treated for chronic pain and respiratory depression is not an issue when a client has been taking opioids for a period of time.

   D. Incorrect: While pulmonary toilet and maintaining as much activity as possible are important in preventing infection and maintaining quality of life, the primary concern is the patient's comfort.

140. Answer is A

   A. **Correct**: The patient receiving palliative care should be permitted to eat whatever he or she desires.

   B. Incorrect: Palliative nutrition should not focus on calories or content. The focus should be on the patient's desires and preferences.

   C. Incorrect: Although the education of the patient should include ways to decrease uncomfortable edema, the patient has choices in palliative care.

   D. Incorrect: Palliative care is providing quality of life according to the wishes of the patient and family. Enteral feeding results in both positive and negative side effects and is not automatically instituted. Patients and families may weigh the benefits and burdens in relation to the patient's quality of life at the time he/she is unable to swallow.

141. Answer is C

   A. Incorrect: In advanced disease, sleeping doesn't necessarily improve the feeling of fatigue.

   B. Incorrect: In advanced disease, the patient is not able to gain weight.

   C. **Correct**: Suffering with poor pain relief can cause the patient to experience fatigue.

   D. Incorrect: Her fatigue could have a basis in depression, but cheering her up and making her laugh would not be an effective intervention for depression or fatigue.

142. The nurse is asking a nursing student to describe the assessment of a client for dyspnea as part of end-of-life care. Which statement by the student indicates understanding of the best method to assess for dyspnea? "I will

A. Auscultate my client's chest."

B. Take my client's respiratory rate."

C. Ask my client about their breathing."

D. Check my client's oxygen saturation rate."

143. The nurse is caring for a client with lung cancer who reports dyspnea. The client has an oxygen saturation level of 94%, a respiratory rate of 26 and is receiving a prescribed continuous intravenous morphine drip. Which of the following actions should the nurse take?

A. Initiate oxygen therapy with a nasal cannula at 5 liters/minute

B. Recommend decreasing the prescribed opioid dosage

C. Suggest an order for oral pharyngeal suctioning

D. Teach the client to use pursed-lip breathing

144. The nurse is teaching the son of a 65-year-old male client with cancer about his father's anorexia. Which statement by the son reassures the nurse that the son understands the teaching and how to best help his father?

A. "We can offer Dad wine before dinner and try to stimulate his appetite."

B. "We need to limit Dad to a high protein diet now."

C. "I need to insist that Dad eat a portion of whatever he is served."

D. "Since Dad isn't eating, it's probably time to put in a feeding tube."

142. Answer is C

   A. Incorrect: See C

   B. Incorrect: See C

   C. **Correct**: Dyspnea is a subjective sensation of breathlessness experienced by the patient and is most appropriately assessed by asking the patient about their symptoms.

   D. Incorrect: See C

143. Answer is D

   A. Incorrect: Since the patient's oxygen saturation level is 94%, there is no indication that administration of oxygen will benefit this patient's symptom.

   B. Incorrect: Opioids can be helpful in relieving the sensation of breathlessness and should not be decreased or discontinued.

   C. Incorrect: There is no indication for suctioning in this patient.

   D. **Correct**: Pursed-lip breathing can be helpful in reducing the sensation of breathlessness.

144. Answer is A

   A. **Correct**: A glass of wine may improve appetite and morale in patients who enjoyed a drink before dinner when they were well.

   B. Incorrect: A high protein diet will not reverse anorexia and cachexia in a patient with advanced cancer.

   C. Incorrect: Forcing patients to eat at the end of life does nothing to improve quality of life.

   D. Incorrect: A decision about a feeding tube is made based on the benefits/burdens of the therapy and the patient's desires and quality of life. A feeding tube will not reverse the course of the patient's disease and may increase discomforts.

145. Which of the following four patients is at the highest risk for developing constipation?

 A. A 48-year-old with metastatic cancer of the spine who has a history of hypercalcemia

 B. A 76-year-old with cancer of the bowel who has begun treatment for Clostridium difficile

 C. An 85-year-old with hepatic encephalopathy who is receiving prescribed neomycin and lactulose

 D. An 90-year-old with lung cancer and hyponatremia

146. The nurse is developing a plan of care for a client with terminal cancer who has a prescribed fentanyl patch and has started to take hydromorphone as a PRN medication. Which goal would be essential to include in the client's plan of care? Client will

 A. Have a pain score of 5 or less as assessed by the nurse

 B. Have usual bowel pattern

 C. Not require PRN meds for breakthrough pain

 D. Not require adjuvant analgesics

147. The nurse is caring for a client in end stage renal disease. The client has no apparent family or support systems. The client is taking prescribed opioid analgesics for pain management yet continues to complain of feeling distressed. The client states, "I wish it would all end." Which action should the nurse take first?

 A. Evaluate the client further for depression

 B. Obtain an order to increase pain medication

 C. Provide diversionary activities

 D. Assess the client's spiritual needs

145. Answer is A

A. **Correct**: Constipation is a symptom of hypercalcemia since hypercalcemia depresses smooth muscle contractility causing decreased intestinal motility. The patient is also most likely on opioid therapy for bone pain, which would significantly increase the risk of constipation as well.

B. Incorrect: Clostridium difficile is an organism that causes diarrhea so a patient who has begun treatment for diarrhea would be unlikely to be at risk for constipation.

C. Incorrect: This patient is receiving medications that would prevent constipation.

D. Incorrect: Hyponatremia is the result of some tumors excreting increased amounts of antidiuretic hormone, which decreases the serum sodium but is not associated with constipation.

146. Answer is B

A. Incorrect: The degree of pain relief that the client desires should be agreed upon with the patient and assessed by the patient's self-report.

B. **Correct**: Management of opioid induced constipation is critical in maintaining the patient's quality of life.

C. Incorrect: While the goal to provide as much pain relief as possible through the scheduled medication (fentanyl) incident pain cannot be predicted.

D. Incorrect: Depending on the underlying etiologies of the patient's pain, adjuvant analgesics may be an important part of the plan of care.

147. Answer is A

A. **Correct**: The patient's suffering may have psychological as well as physical components that should be assessed and treated if appropriate.

B. Incorrect: Increasing pain medication is not appropriate because the patient is not complaining of pain.

C. Incorrect: Diversion or distraction can be useful in some situations but will not be helpful when a patient is ruminating about their situation.

D. Incorrect: While the patient's spiritual needs should also be assessed, depression should be assessed first.

148. The home health nurse is caring for a client at the end of life who has a recent history of constipation. The nurse should assess the client for which indicator of fecal impaction?

   A. Foul smelling diarrhea

   B. Sudden onset of liquid stool

   C. Fatty looking stools

   D. Blood and mucous strands in stool

149. The nurse has conducted a staff development in-service on assessing the patient who experiences dyspnea at the end of life. Which statement by a participant following the in-service would require the nurse to question the participant's understanding of dyspnea?

   A. "I will assess jugular vein pressure on a patient who reports dyspnea."

   B. "I need to utilize the patient's description to determine the degree of dyspnea."

   C. "I will ask the patient how the dyspnea is affecting their lifestyle."

   D. "Dyspnea is present only in advanced disease."

150. To prevent dehydration in the advanced cancer patient prone to hypercalcemia, which of the following fluids is recommended?

   A. Broth

   B. Water

   C. Carbonated beverages

   D. Fruit juice

148.   Answer is B

    A.   Incorrect: Foul smelling diarrhea may be indicative of an infection but not constipation.

    B.   **Correct**: Sudden onset of liquid stool may indicate oozing around an impaction.

    C.   Incorrect: Fatty looking stools may be indicative of other gastrointestinal problems, but not impaction.

    D.   Incorrect: Blood and mucous strands are not indicative of impaction.

149.   Answer is D

    A.   Incorrect: Assessment of JVP would be part of the overall physical examination of patients with respiratory problems.

    B.   Incorrect: The patient's description is the most important since dyspnea is the sensation of breathlessness experienced by the client.

    C.   Incorrect: When assessing the patient's experience with this symptom it is important to note the impact on lifestyle and activities of daily living.

    D.   **Correct**: Dyspnea may be present in cardiac and respiratory conditions in earlier stages.

150.   Answer is A

    A.   **Correct**: Broth is high in sodium and can help maintain extracellular fluid balance by replacing both sodium and water.

    B.   Incorrect: Water does not contain the sodium necessary to assist in maintaining fluid balance.

    C.   Incorrect: Carbonated beverages are not indicated in preventing dehydration in hypercalcemia.

    D.   Incorrect: Fruit juice does not contain the sodium necessary to assist in maintaining fluid balance.

151. For the patient who has advanced dementia, the priority therapeutic intervention is

    A. Keep TV on to distract patient from wandering

    B. Explain every procedure in detail

    C. Anticipate safety needs

    D. Encourage frequent naps

Care of the Patient and Family

152. The nurse is performing an admission assessment of a client with amyotrophic lateral sclerosis (ALS). Which principle should the nurse use to determine the priorities for care of this patient?

    A. The control of symptoms is essential before assessment of other dimensions

    B. The interdisciplinary team should determine which dimension is most important

    C. The client and family should decide which dimension is critical to them

    D. The nurse should identify the most important dimension after assessment

153. The nurse is caring for a 48-year-old woman recently diagnosed with breast cancer. The client is married and has 3 small children. What is the best time to begin a spiritual assessment?

    A. When the patient enters the healthcare system

    B. After chemotherapy is initiated

    C. Once the patient asks for spiritual support

    D. As soon as the client begins to deteriorate

151.   Answer is C

   A.   Incorrect: Individuals with advanced dementia should have minimal stimulation.

   B.   Incorrect: Healthcare workers should use simple words and explanations with the demented patient.

   C.   **Correct**: Safety is a major concern and should be a priority with demented patients. Supervision, minimal stimulation and discouraging sleep during daytime hours to maximize night safety.

   D.   Incorrect: Naps should be discouraged at any time of the day.

Care of the Patient and Family

152.   Answer is C

   A.   Incorrect: While the control of symptoms is important, the nurse must find out which issues are most important to the patient and family at that time.

   B.   Incorrect: While the team is involved in care planning with the patient and family, the preferences and needs of the patient and the family drive the care plan.

   C.   **Correct**: The nurse needs to assess the patient and family's primary concerns.

   D.   Incorrect: See A

153.   Answer is A

   A.   **Correct**: Spiritual assessment should be part of the initial assessment that helps to guide and direct care.

   B.   Incorrect: Spiritual assessment should be done prior to developing the plan of care for the patient.

   C.   Incorrect: Once the client has asked for spiritual support, she may have been suffering for some period and could have benefited from early identification of needs.

   D.   Incorrect: The client should have the opportunity to address spiritual issues before physical condition impedes ability.

154. The nurse is caring for a client from Cambodia who has terminal lung cancer. The client is reluctant to discuss the illness. Which action should the nurse take?

   A. Remind the client that it is important to talk about the illness

   B. Allow the client to remain in denial by not discussing the cancer

   C. Ask the family about their beliefs regarding full disclosure

   D. Refer the client to a mental health professional for evaluation

155. The nurse is teaching a nursing student how to perform a cultural assessment for patients at the end of life. Which statement by the student indicates a correct understanding of cultural assessment?

   A. "The best strategy for evaluating sexual orientation is to ask clients if they are heterosexual or homosexual."

   B. "To assess spirituality, questions regarding religious affiliation and religious practices are generally sufficient."

   C. "Financial status is a sensitive topic and should be assessed by the social worker."

   D. "Ethnic identity varies within ethnic groups, so ask clients how strongly they identify with a particular group."

156. The nurse is caring for a client admitted to the hospital with a diagnosis of colon cancer. The client speaks only Spanish, the nurse speaks only English and some family members speak both. The nurse wants to discuss pain management with the patient. Which approach is most appropriate?

   A. Request that a hospital interpreter meet with the patient and family

   B. Ask a family member to serve as the primary spokesperson for the patient

   C. Solicit one of the patient's close friends to serve as an informal translator

   D. Find a member of the patient's church or social circle to serve as interpreter

154. Answer is C

    A. Incorrect: Talking about the illness may not be valued by this client. The nurse should, however, make attempts to assess the need for psychological or spiritual interventions.

    B. Incorrect: This would not be an appropriate action until further assessment is completed.

    C. **Correct**: This would be part of continued assessment of the patient and family's needs and preferences.

    D. Incorrect: See B

155. Answer is D

    A. Incorrect: This answer is too prescriptive; an open-ended question about sexuality or sexual issues of concern is preferable.

    B. Incorrect: Again, questions regarding religious affiliation and practices may be too prescriptive and do not allow for full exploration of spiritual issues not limited by religion.

    C. Incorrect: Financial status can be assessed by any competent health professional if it is relevant to the development of the plan of care and is approached sensitively.

    D. **Correct**: Assumptions should not be made about ethnic and/or cultural identity and practices without validating the patient's unique identity and beliefs.

156. Answer is A

    A. **Correct**: Healthcare agencies receiving federal funds are required to provide interpretive services for clients speaking commonly encountered foreign languages at no charge to the patient. This is the best option and meets federal guidelines.

    B. Incorrect: Federal guidance from the Office of Civil Rights states that family members cannot be required to serve as interpreters unless the client specifically requests a family member to be used in this capacity. The client must be informed that an interpreter from the hospital is available free of charge.

    C. Incorrect: See B. To ensure appropriate care and communication, the best possible interpreter should be found who is trained in medical terminology, fluent in both languages and knows the ethics of interpreting and HIPAA regulations. In emergency situations, informal translators may be a necessity.

    D. Incorrect: See B and C

157. During the weekly hospice interdisciplinary team meeting, a nurse reports concern regarding a woman she assessed during a bereavement visit. The woman's husband died four months ago. The family is Greek Orthodox and the nurse is concerned that the wife may be depressed because she refuses to take part in social activities outside the home. The most important reason for the nurse to bring issues/concerns to the interdisciplinary team is so the team members can

   A. Help the nurse cope with her concerns

   B. Offer guidance in cultural assessments and plan of care

   C. Provide resources to increase her socialization

   D. Offer suggestions to get the wife to seek treatment

158. The nurse is orienting to palliative care and is identifying necessary learning activities. In order to provide culturally sensitive care to those at the end of life, one of the nurse's earliest orientation tasks should be to

   A. Identify one's own cultural background and values

   B. Evaluate the cultural beliefs of co-workers

   C. Learn to predict how various races deal with end-of-life issues

   D. Enroll in a diversity training program

159. In palliative care the nurse cares for people of many cultures. When conversing with persons of another culture the nurse should

   A. Use the patient's first name to establish warm rapport

   B. Act as if the patient is fully informed of the diagnosis and prognosis

   C. Speak primarily to the translator rather than the patient or family

   D. Determine who makes decisions for the patient and family

157. Answer is B

    A. Incorrect: The role of the team is to help provide a multidisciplinary perspective in assessment and developing the plan of care.

    B. **Correct**: See A

    C. Incorrect: An intervention needs to be based on a thorough interdisciplinary assessment and there may be alternative explanations for her refusal to take part in social activities (formal period of mourning, cultural tradition). Assumptions should not be made before the assessment is complete. Additional team members may need to become involved.

    D. Incorrect: See C

158. Answer is A

    A. **Correct**: The nurse should be aware of his/her own background and values so that he/she will be more able to recognize biases.

    B. Incorrect: While the nurse may come to know some of the cultural beliefs and values of co-workers over time, this is not a primary concern.

    C. Incorrect: While the nurse may become aware of some differences in approaches to end-of-life care by ethnicity or race, this knowledge should be used to be more sensitive and open to the differences rather than trying to predict behavior. Each person must receive individualized assessment and care and assumptions should not be made about their needs and preferences based on their race or ethnicity.

    D. Incorrect: While this may be of benefit to the nurse, this is not the best answer.

159. Answer is D

    A. Incorrect: The nurse should not assume familiarity with a patient until he/she has determined what the patient prefers to be called.

    B. Incorrect: The nurse should not assume that the patient and/or family desired full disclosure from their healthcare team.

    C. Incorrect: Even when using an interpreter, the nurse should speak to the person he/she is trying to communicate with.

    D. **Correct**: An assessment regarding family communication and decision-making is important in order to complete a comprehensive assessment and determine appropriate interventions.

160. To the culturally sensitive palliative care nurse "cultural competence" is most correctly defined as

    A. Knowing general facts about other ethnic and cultural groups

    B. Sharing the nurse's own cultural and ethnic beliefs with patients

    C. Performing skillful and sensitive cultural assessments on patients

    D. Adapting the plan of care to be congruent with the client's culture

161. Which question is the **LEAST** appropriate during a spiritual assessment?

    A. "What church do you attend?"

    B. "Are spiritual beliefs important in your life?"

    C. "What aspect of your faith gives your life most meaning?"

    D. "How would you like me to address spirituality in your care?"

162. The nurse is caring for a client who just had surgery that revealed stage IV ovarian cancer. The client does not know her diagnosis. Which action should the nurse take in preparation for the client to be told her diagnosis?

    A. Make sure all team members are able to be present

    B. Find a neutral, non-threatening location in which to tell the news

    C. Make sure that appropriate medications for anxiety are prescribed

    D. Find out how much the patient/family want to know

160. Answer is D

    A. Incorrect: Knowing general facts does not translate into culturally competent behavior.

    B. Incorrect: Cultural sensitivity is being aware of one's own beliefs and not allowing them to have an undue effect on the care provided.

    C. Incorrect: Providing skillful and sensitive cultural assessments is a component on being culturally competent but would be inadequate unless the nurse was able to use the assessment to develop a meaningful care plan.

    D. **Correct**: Cultural competence is the provision of care that fits with the patient's cultural background and requires knowledge of one's own beliefs/values, skillful assessment and executing a plan of care that incorporates this awareness and skill.

161. Answer is A

    A. **Correct**: Religious practice is not as important or relevant as overall spirituality. Asking the question in this way assumes that the patient attends church, which may be insensitive for non-Christians or people who do not actively participate in organized religion.

    B. Incorrect: This is not the least appropriate question but it is not the best either as it is a yes/no question and will not lead the patient to elaborate on their faith or beliefs.

    C. Incorrect: This question gives the patient an opportunity to think and express their belief.

    D. Incorrect: This question provides information for the nurse in terms of what interventions will be preferred, if any.

162. Answer is D

    A. Incorrect: Not all team members need to be present in order for the discussion to take place.

    B. Incorrect: The patient who is recovering from surgery will probably not have options of moving from the hospital be/room.

    C. Incorrect: Anxiety should not be assumed.

    D. **Correct**: Before making any disclosure, an appropriate assessment should be made of how much the patient/family want to know.

163. The nurse is working with a nursing student in caring for a 5-year-old boy with a brain tumor. The child is dying and the student is concerned about how to relate to the client and family. Which statement by the student indicates the best understanding of communicating in this situation?

   A. "I will ask the parents to determine how the child is coping with his illness."

   B. "I will try to understand the parent's and child's perception of the illness."

   C. "I will offer positive encouragement to the child and the family."

   D. "I will determine if the child and family have unmet spiritual needs."

164. In preparing to discuss bad news with a patient, the palliative care nurse should

   A. Speak from the heart, without rehearsal to convey sincerity

   B. Determine what the patient and family already know

   C. Presume that patients want and need to be told the truth

   D. Be prepared to give advice about future treatment options

165. The nurse is caring for a man with advanced prostate cancer. He has been told that his therapy is not working. He asks the nurse, "Why is this happening to me?" What is the nurse's most appropriate response?

   A. "I don't know. I wish I had an answer for you, but I don't."

   B. "Perhaps you're being tested and this will make you a stronger person."

   C. "I'll ask the doctor to more fully explain the disease process."

   D. "If I were you, I'd explore additional therapies and treatment options."

163. Answer is B

  A. Incorrect: It would be inappropriate to ask the parents to assess their own child's needs at this time in the illness.

  B. **Correct**: Assessment and understanding through quiet observation and presence will assist the student nurse in feeling comfortable and providing emotional support to the family.

  C. Incorrect: Positive encouragement in the face of grief and loss may not be appropriate.

  D. Incorrect: See B

164. Answer is B

  A. Incorrect: Because this is such a sensitive topic, the nurse may need to choose words carefully and prepare in advance.

  B. **Correct**: Assessment is always the best place to start and determining what is known will be helpful in knowing where to start.

  C. Incorrect: Nothing should be presumed, everything should be assessed in advance, including patients' preferences regarding the degree of disclosure.

  D. Incorrect: This would be beyond the scope of nursing practice.

165. Answer is A

  A. **Correct**: The patient is not actually asking for the nurse to explain why, but to validate that there is no easy explanation.

  B. Incorrect: This would be an inappropriate response because it could be perceived negatively and create guilt in the individual. The response feels like the nurse is imposing beliefs on the patient.

  C. Incorrect: See A

  D. Incorrect: At this point in the disease process, it is more helpful to be present with the patient and supportive as he struggles with accepting the change in his prognosis.

166. The nurse is trying to initiate a conversation with a dying patient about end-of-life issues. The patient, usually talkative with the nurse, is unusually quiet and prefers not to talk. Which reason for the patient's silence would be a maladaptive response?

A. The patient is in denial about the seriousness of the disease

B. The patient's need for information has been met by someone else

C. The patient needs additional time to consider the diagnosis and prognosis

D. The patient withdraws and will not discuss the bad news with his healthcare team or family

167. The nurse is speaking with the family member of a patient in the Neuro ICU. The nurse employs attentive listening to encourage dialogue. The nurse best demonstrates attentive listening by

A. Interrupting the conversation to clarify what the family member means

B. Using non-verbal signals such as nodding one's head and eye contact

C. Periodically giving a summary of what the family member has said

D. Using yes/no questions to enhance the flow of conversation

168. For the past week, the nurse has been caring for a client in the advanced stages of HIV/AIDS. The nurse hopes to find time to assess the client's emotional and spiritual needs. The nurse's first action to open the communication process should be to

A. Find out if the client feels like talking

B. Sit close to the client to demonstrate empathy

C. Move the client to a setting that ensures privacy

D. Pray with or witness to the patient

166. Answer is D

    A. Incorrect: Limited denial can be an adaptive response.

    B. Incorrect: If the patient's needs are met, silence would not be maladaptive.

    C. Incorrect: If the patient needs more time to process before responding, silence would not be maladaptive.

    D. **Correct**: Withdrawal may be a sign of depression that may require further assessment and treatment.

167. Answer is B

    A. Incorrect: Interrupting is not listening.

    B. **Correct**: Using non-verbal signals and open body language are the best ways to demonstrate active and attentive listening and encourage the flow of dialogue and discussion.

    C. Incorrect: While this answer is not incorrect, it is not the best way to demonstrate active listening. This technique is most helpful in validating the family's statements.

    D. Incorrect: Yes/no questions are closed rather than open-ended and do not assist the flow of conversation or active listening.

168. Answer is A

    A. **Correct**: Nursing process begins with good assessment; does the patient feel like engaging in this conversation today?

    B. Incorrect: While sitting close may convey empathy, this is not the best first action.

    C. Incorrect: While this may be an appropriate intervention, it is not the best first action.

    D. Incorrect: Unsolicited prayer or preaching without a request from the patient is clearly inappropriate prior to completion of an assessment that establishes the patient's preferences for spiritual care.

169. An 85-year-old client with end-stage heart disease arrives unconscious at the emergency department after sustaining her third myocardial infarction. The physician has told the daughter that without putting her on ventilatory support, her mother could die today. The nurse finds the daughter crying by the client's bedside. Which intervention by the nurse is most appropriate in communicating with this family member?

    A. Ask the daughter if she would like to reconsider treatment

    B. Talk to the physician about moving the client to a unit with more privacy

    C. Remain present with the daughter, using silence to impart comfort

    D. Assure the daughter that she doesn't need to stay with her mother

170. The hospice nurse is making a bereavement visit to the 35-year-old daughter and primary caregiver of a female client who died 3 months ago. The daughter reports she is experiencing mild breathlessness, loss of appetite and difficulty concentrating. The nurse should recognize that the daughter is experiencing

    A. A normal grief reaction

    B. A complicated grief reaction

    C. An abnormal grief reaction

    D. A dysfunctional grief reaction

171. The nurse is caring for a 65-year-old male client who has just died. In planning for follow-up bereavement care, which person is at risk for disenfranchised grief?

    A. The daughter who lives in a different state

    B. The son who was with the client when he died

    C. The ex-wife of the patient who lives nearby

    D. The 16-year-old grandchild of the client

169. Answer is C

    A. Incorrect: The nurse is assuming that she knows why the daughter is crying and jumps to an intervention without adequately assessing.

    B. Incorrect: See A

    C. **Correct**: Remaining present with the daughter gives the nurse an opportunity to provide comfort, but also opens the door for the daughter to share her concerns and grief. This may provide the nurse with more assessment data from which to derive other supportive interventions.

    D. Incorrect: See A

170. Answer is A

    A. **Correct**: The mild symptoms the daughter is experiencing can all be attributed to grief. However, if the symptoms persisted or increased, physical causes should be ruled out.

    B. Incorrect: There are no indications of a complicated grief reaction.

    C. Incorrect: There are no indications of an abnormal grief reaction

    D. Incorrect: There are no indications of a dysfunctional grief reaction

171. Answer is C

    A. Incorrect: See C

    B. Incorrect: See C

    C. **Correct**: Disenfranchised grief is the experience of loss that cannot be openly acknowledged, publicly mourned or socially supported. The ex-wife may not be welcome at mourning events or have an opportunity to express the grief in a public way with the support of others who understand her grief.

    D. Incorrect: See C

172. The nurse is talking with the wife of a client who died recently. Which statement by the nurse is most helpful?

   A. "I know exactly how you are feeling."

   B. "It must be hard to accept that this has happened."

   C. "His suffering is over. He's in a better place now."

   D. "I'm here for you. Call me if you need anything."

173. The hospice nurse is caring for the family of a man who died several days ago after a long illness. His wife is concerned that their 9-year-old son has become withdrawn and is easily angered. Which action is most appropriate for the nurse?

   A. Recommend the boy be referred to a specialist for complicated grief reaction

   B. Suggest to the mother that the boy be excused from his usual activities

   C. Give permission and opportunities for the boy to express feelings of loss

   D. Provide information about death to the boy by telling stories rather than giving facts

174. The new nurse is caring for a number of patients and family members who are facing loss or death. In speaking with them about grief, the nurse correctly conveys that grief

   A. Is an orderly process with predictable stages of work to be done

   B. Begins before a loss or death, as people consider a pending loss

   C. Lasts a year or less, at which time survivors should be able to move on

   D. Includes personal feelings that are universal and understood by everyone

172. Answer is B

    A. Incorrect: The nurse does not know exactly how the wife is feeling and this can be interpreted to be an insensitive statement.

    B. **Correct**: This is an open statement that empathizes with the wife without describing the experience for her. It provides an opportunity for the wife to respond without demanding a response in the form of a question.

    C. Incorrect: While it may be comforting to the wife if the patient suffered to know it has ended, but the nurse cannot assume that the wife believes he is in a better place now or that his suffering has ended. The nurse should first assess the wife's beliefs and concerns.

    D. Incorrect: This statement indicates inappropriate understanding of the professional role of the nurse and appropriate boundaries.

173. Answer is C

    A. Incorrect: Based on the case information, there is no indication of a complicated grief reaction at this time.

    B. Incorrect: This assumes an intervention without an appropriate assessment and opportunity to find out what the son's feelings are.

    C. **Correct**: The nurse and the wife need to provide presence and availability and space for the son to be able to express his feelings of loss more directly than through his behavior.

    D. Incorrect: This is more appropriate anticipatory information before the death than after.

174. Answer is B

    A. Incorrect: Grief is not orderly and while there are stages or tasks, they are not predictable and the bereaved can move back and forth between them.

    B. **Correct**: This is a true statement. Grief begins in response to an anticipated loss.

    C. Incorrect: There is no definitive time period associated with grief. It is individual.

    D. Incorrect: While grief and loss are part of the human condition, individual reactions to loss are not universal or understood by everyone.

175. The nurse is caring for a 55-year-old female client with metastatic breast cancer. During a home visit, the nurse finds the client's 22-year-old daughter weeping at the kitchen table. The daughter explains that she just realized that her mother will not be alive when she gets married or has children of her own. The best nursing intervention at the time is

   A. Educate about signs and symptoms of disease progression

   B. Foster hope by stressing that prognosis is difficult to predict

   C. Provide therapeutic presence and practice active listening

   D. Advise the daughter to focus more on the present than the future

176. The wife of a recently deceased patient states: "Last night I thought I heard him say 'Good night, Honey' just like he always did. Do you think I am going crazy?" The most helpful response by the nurse will be

   A. "You might want some extra support accepting your husband's death. I'll have the doctor make a referral to a psychologist."

   B. "Many people have a similar experience of seeing or hearing the one who has died. You must miss him saying 'good night'."

   C. "Many people believe that the spirit of one who has died visits their loved ones after death. Do you believe that your husband's spirit is returning? Why?"

   D. "That must be frightening for you. Do you have a friend or relative who can stay with you so that you are not alone?"

177. The nurse is orienting new staff to a clinical unit that provides palliative care. A new employee asks what "grief" is exactly. The nurse correctly defines grief as the

   A. Emotional response to a loss

   B. Outward, social expression of a loss

   C. Depression felt after a loss

   D. Loss of a possession or loved one

175. Answer is C

    A. Incorrect: The daughter is expressing anticipatory grief and does not need information at this time. She needs support.

    B. Incorrect: Hope should be supported for the current day and what the daughter can have with the mother in the time remaining, not fostering unrealistic hope regarding prognosis.

    C. **Correct**: Providing therapeutic presence and active listening are appropriate interventions for supporting the daughter, as she is grieving.

    D. Incorrect: This may be an appropriate intervention at a different point in time, but not while the daughter is in immediate emotional distress

176. Answer is B

    A. Incorrect: There is no rationale for a referral to a psychologist as the behavior being experienced is a normal grief reaction.

    B. **Correct**: The nurse validates the normality of the wife's experience and gives her an opportunity to discuss her feelings of loss.

    C. Incorrect: In this statement and question the nurse is introducing inappropriate material unrelated to an assessment of the wife's beliefs and/or values.

    D. Incorrect: This statement may increase the wife's fears and does not validate the normality of the experience.

177. Answer is A

    A. **Correct**: This is the definition of grief.

    B. Incorrect: This is the definition of mourning.

    C. Incorrect: Grief is not the same as depression.

    D. Incorrect: Loss is not the same as grief, which is the emotional experience associated with loss.

178. The nurse is caring for the family of a client who died two months ago. During a home visit, the wife of the deceased states "It's just so typical, him leaving me to fend for myself. He was always so selfish." The nurse recognizes that the task of grief that the wife is most likely dealing with is

   A. Working through the pain of the loss

   B. Readjusting and adapting to the new role

   C. Reorganizing and restructuring family systems

   D. Reinvesting in new relationships

179. The emergency department nurse is speaking with the sister of a male client who died after suffering fatal injuries in a car accident. In order to plan for bereavement follow-up for the client's family, it is important that the nurse assess all of the following **EXCEPT**

   A. Family support systems

   B. Spiritual belief systems

   C. Concurrent stressors

   D. Advance directives

180. The nurse has been caring for a Latino client with advanced obstructive lung disease for the past several weeks. The client's family has been at the bedside daily, with one member spending the night throughout the client's hospital stay. In assessing cultural beliefs and practices related to death and dying for the client and family, it is necessary that the nurse should take into consideration all of the following factors **EXCEPT**

   A. Aspects of spirituality, traditions, rites and rituals

   B. The age of the client and family members

   C. How long the client has been in this country

   D. Specific beliefs about pain, suffering, and death

178. Answer is A

    A. **Correct**: Working through the pain of loss includes working through anger.

    B. Incorrect: The wife is not showing evidence of readjustment or adaptation at this stage.

    C. Incorrect: The wife is not talking about reorganizing or restructuring family systems.

    D. Incorrect: The wife is not yet reinvesting in new relationships.

179. Answer is D

    A. Incorrect: Assessment of family support systems is important in determining who may be at risk for complicated grief and developing an appropriate plan of care.

    B. Incorrect: Spiritual belief systems are part of an appropriate bereavement assessment.

    C. Incorrect: Knowing the family's other stressors is important in understanding the risk for complicated grief and developing an appropriate plan of care.

    D. **Correct**: Advance directives are no longer relevant after the patient has died.

180. Answer is C

    A. Incorrect: Assessing these variables is an important part of a comprehensive assessment that enables an individualized plan of care.

    B. Incorrect: This is an important part of the assessment as developmental tasks related to grief vary by age.

    C. **Correct**: How long the client has been in this country is not relevant to developing a plan of care. What is relevant are the patient and family's beliefs, values, culture and traditions.

    D. Incorrect: Knowing the patient and family's beliefs about pain, suffering and death will help guide education and psychosocial and spiritual support.

181. The parents of a terminally ill 7-month-old child are at the bedside when the child dies. The nurse supports the family's initial grief reactions by initiating all of the following interventions **EXCEPT**

   A. Offer the parents an opportunity to hold the child

   B. Support inclusion of siblings in death rituals

   C. Wrap the child securely in a blanket

   D. Avoid remarks regarding the child's life

182. Mr. Able is 70 years old and newly admitted to the hospice program in a long-term care facility. He no longer recognizes his family, is bed bound and presents with extreme rigidity of all extremities. As you initiate the plan of care, all of the following choices are appropriate interventions **EXCEPT**

   A. Create an atmosphere with limited stimulation

   B. Teach and/or reinforce with facility staff the importance of regular assessments of skin integrity

   C. Frequent and gentle stimulation (i.e., touch and music)

   D. Encourage family to remain/become involved with care

183. Mr. Able, from the previous question, becomes less agitated, but claims to see his deceased wife and mother and hears them asking him to "come home." The family is upset and has asked you to sedate him. What is your response?

   A. Contact the physician and ask for an order for haloperidol

   B. Restrain Mr. Able

   C. Call the chaplain to address the spiritual pain

   D. Assure the family this is normal, nearing death awareness

181.   Answer is D

   A.   Incorrect: This is an appropriate intervention that may help the parents in accepting the loss and let-
        ting go of the child.

   B.   Incorrect: Siblings should be included in the rituals surrounding death and mourning as it can help
        channel their grief and provide them the structure and support they need when experiencing this
        loss.

   C.   Incorrect: This is an appropriate preparation of the body.

   D.   **Correct**: It is not necessary to avoid remarks regarding the child's life. The parents and family will
        want to remember their child's life and this can be validating for them.

182.   Answer is C

   A.   Incorrect: This would be an important option. A quiet atmosphere with limited stimulation would be
        preferred in this situation.

   B.   Incorrect: Skin care is a priority in this case due to the extreme rigidity of his extremities.

   C.   **Correct**: While music therapy can sometimes be soothing, in this case, frequent stimulation would
        not be advisable so this could be eliminated in patients with neurologic involvement.

   D.   Incorrect: We seek to involve the family whenever possible so we would not want to eliminate this
        choice.

183.   Answer is D

   A.   Incorrect: There would be no reason to sedate Mr. Able. His family needs reassurance and support as
        well as education to help them understand what is happening.

   B.   Incorrect: Restraints would be totally inappropriate and may cause more agitation.

   C.   Incorrect: While there is a spiritual aspect to this situation, the action of choice is to recognize the
        normalcy of what is happening.

   D.   **Correct**: Near death awareness is associated with dreams or visions of deceased people, God or
        heaven. One needs to assess the special awareness, needs and communications of the dying and
        encourage verbalization without judgment or interpretation. One should encourage the family to be
        present and share important messages with patient, listen for meaning or meaningful experiences,
        distinguish between "confusion" and symbolic communication (i.e. "going home" may not refer to
        an unrealistic possibility, it may mean an after life to the patient).

184. The process of psychological, social, and somatic reactions to a perceived future loss is known as

    A. Mourning

    B. Grief

    C. Bereavement

    D. Anticipatory grief

185. The cultural response to having suffered a loss is

    A. Mourning

    B. Grief

    C. Anticipatory grief

    D. Bereavement

186. When a patient is comatose, the nurse should

    A. Speak to the patient as if he/she were not there

    B. Speak to the patient as if he/she can hear

    C. Do not speak in the room at all

    D. Speak only to family members

187. The state of having suffered a loss is

    A. Mourning

    B. Grief

    C. Bereavement

    D. Anticipatory grief

184. Answer is D

    A. Incorrect: Mourning is the cultural response to having suffered a loss.

    B. Incorrect: Grief is the process of psychological, social, and somatic reactions to a perceived loss.

    C. Incorrect: Bereavement is the state of having suffered a loss.

    D. **Correct**: This is the definition of anticipatory grief.

185. Answer is A

    A. **Correct**: This is the definition of mourning.

    B. Incorrect: Grief is the process of psychological, social, and somatic reactions to a perceived loss.

    C. Incorrect: Anticipatory grief is the process of psychological, social, and somatic reactions to a perceived future loss.

    D. Incorrect: Bereavement is the state of having suffered a loss.

186. Answer is B

    A. Incorrect: Dying persons can hear especially familiar sounds therefore family and healthcare workers should be encouraged to continue to speak to the patient in soft soothing tones.

    B. **Correct**: One should continue to speak as if the patient hears since it is believed the sense of hearing is the last sense the patient loses.

    C. Incorrect: Patients are comforted by familiar sounds—it is important to continue to speak softly.

    D. Incorrect: Patient can still hear.

187. Answer is C

    A. Incorrect: Mourning is the cultural response to having suffered a loss.

    B. Incorrect: Grief is the process of psychological, social, and somatic reactions to a perceived loss.

    C. **Correct**: This is the definition of bereavement.

    D. Incorrect: Anticipatory grief is the process of psychological, social, and somatic reactions to a perceived future loss.

188. Spiritual care of the hospice patient and family

    A. Is provided in accordance with the religion of the hospice chaplain

    B. Is only provided by a hospice staff member

    C. Is provided to every patient and family admitted to hospice care

    D. Identifies and strives to relieve the spiritual suffering of the patient and family

189. The extent and duration of grief

    A. Are pretty much the same from person to person

    B. Vary considerably from person to person

    C. Differ considerably between men and women

    D. Are the same when death is expected and planned for

190. For grief to be pathological, it must

    A. Be more than a year in duration

    B. Affect most aspects of the person's life

    C. Be preceded by depression

    D. Grief cannot be pathological

188. Answer is D

    A. Incorrect: Spiritual care must be provided according to the patient's religion of choice.

    B. Incorrect: Spiritual care can be provided by any one known to the patient.

    C. Incorrect: Spiritual care is provided according to the wishes of the patient. If they do not wish to have spiritual counseling, it is not required.

    D. **Correct**: Spiritual care is intended to relieve the spiritual suffering of the patient and family.

189. Answer is B

    A. Incorrect: Grief is not the same with each individual; many variations exist.

    B. **Correct**: Grief has a very individual response.

    C. Incorrect: Grief does have gender variability in some individuals but have many other differences as well.

    D. Incorrect: The extent and duration of grief has multiple variables.

190. Answer is B

    A. Incorrect: One aspect alone does not describe pathologic grief.

    B. **Correct**: Pathological grief is complicated and affects all aspects of the individual's life.

    C. Incorrect: Clinical depression is not a necessary antecedent of grief. Grief is the response to a loss and is not necessarily preceded by depression.

    D. Incorrect: Grief can indeed be pathologic.

191. Sarah, a 4-year-old whose mother recently died, is able to play with her friends, laugh, and enjoy her toys. Sarah is

    A. Obviously depressed

    B. Showing disrespect for her mother's memory

    C. Grieving normally for a child her age

    D. Is in need of intensive grief counseling

192. Which of the following is **NOT** a principle of adult learning?

    A. Collaborating

    B. Memorization

    C. Critically reflective thinking

    D. Learning for action

193. Appropriate instructions for a 7-year-old hospice or palliative care patient may include the following statements **EXCEPT**

    A. "Drink one glass of water with your pills."

    B. "Ask for help when going to the bathroom."

    C. "Death is like going to sleep."

    D. "Tell me when and where it hurts."

194. In hospice, the patient and family are considered the unit of care. Which statement most accurately describes dying patients and their families?

    A. A search for meaning and purpose in life is a common experience for dying patients and their families

    B. Dying patients and their families are too consumed with financial problems ever to think about spiritual concerns

    C. Dying patients and their families have little to fear because hospice takes care of everything

    D. The same care plan can be used for all families because their needs are the same

191. Answer is C

    A. Incorrect: There may be intense periods separated by long intervals where they apparently are not affected by the loss.

    B. Incorrect: Sarah's behavior is normal and not a sign of disrespect for her mother's memory.

    C. **Correct**: Sarah's behavior is normal for her age.

    D. Incorrect: Sarah's grasp of concepts related to death, time, and permanence are limited and children her age often see death as temporary.

192. Answer is B

    A. Incorrect: Collaborating is a principle of adult learning.

    B. **Correct**: This is not a principle of adult learning. Principles include collaborating, critically reflective thinking, learning for action, learning in a participative environment, empowering learners, dialoguing in the educational process, and self directed learning.

    C. Incorrect: Critically reflective thinking is a principle of adult learning.

    D. Incorrect: Learning for action is a principle of adult learning.

193. Answer is C

    A. Incorrect: This is appropriate instruction for a 7-year-old.

    B. Incorrect: See A.

    C. **Correct**: This statement would not be appropriate; it may reinforce the idea that death is temporary which is common in younger children.

    D. Incorrect: See A.

194. Answer is A

    A. **Correct**: Patients and families search for meaning of the individual's life and seek a purpose during the dying phase.

    B. Incorrect: Although financial concerns should never be minimized, the focus of the dying patient and their families is not the financial concerns.

    C. Incorrect: Hospice provides guidance and assistance to the patient and family but does not take over family functioning.

    D. Incorrect: Every care plan is individualized therefore no two are alike.

195. E. L. is an 11-year-old Cambodian boy who suffered an anoxic event five years previous to the admission. He has been living in a chronic vegetative state since the injury. Recently he has been developing recurrent pneumonias. The family is now questioning his quality of life. What information about Cambodian culture should the treatment team factor into the care plan?

    A. What role does healthcare take in healing

    B. What is the role of the family in making healthcare decisions

    C. What do Cambodians believe about withdrawing of treatment such as feeding tubes, antibiotics, etc.?

    D. All of the above

196. When the patient dies in the home, the Schedule II drugs are

    A. Property of the hospice

    B. Disposed of by the nurse with a witness present

    C. Returned to the hospice or pharmacy for credit

    D. Property of the family

Indicators of Imminent Dying

197. Mrs. M has end-stage illness, has lost 20% of her body weight and is experiencing increasing weakness. The best nutritional approach for Mrs. M. would be

    A. A trial of hydration

    B. Insertion of a feeding tube for enteral nutrition

    C. Eating on demand, not on a fixed schedule

    D. A dietary consult to reverse the weight loss

195.   Answer is D

    A. Incorrect: This is one aspect to factor into the plan.

    B. Incorrect: The role of the family is very important, but not the only factor.

    C. Incorrect: Withdrawing treatment must be explored with the Cambodian culture along with the other factors.

    D. **Correct**: Good palliative care takes into account the role of health and how it is defined in that culture, as well as the family, including how they make decisions and the extent of technology they want used. Some cultures use healers rather than Western medicine. In addition, some do not want the body invaded when someone is close to death. The palliative care team needs to elicit this information in order to deliver respectful care.

196.   Answer is B

    A. Incorrect: These drugs do not belong to the hospice.

    B. **Correct**: The drugs should be discarded by the nurse who is responsible for medication management and witnessed by a second individual.

    C. Incorrect: There is no guarantee that the medications have not been altered in some manner and cannot legally be returned to the pharmacy.

    D. Incorrect: These medications should be disposed of by the medical professional responsible for medication management with a witness.

Indicators of Imminent Dying

197.   Answer is C

    A. Incorrect: Weight loss and weakness do not necessarily mean that Mrs. M. is dehydrated.

    B. Incorrect: Artificial feeding can increase pain, discomfort and other complications without significant benefit.

    C. **Correct**: While maintaining weight or a level of caloric intake is not achievable in patients nearing death, patients can still enjoy eating and drinking for comfort and social pleasure.

    D. Incorrect: Reversing weight loss is not a realistic goal at end-stage.

198. Which of the following is the best description of spiritual issues at the end of life?

    A. Primarily related to religious beliefs and rituals

    B. Characterized by "why" questions

    C. Primarily related to feeling out of control

    D. Best delegated to community clergy

199. Which of the following requires immediate intervention for patient distress?

    A. Mild dyspnea

    B. Cheyne-Stokes breathing pattern

    C. Periods of apnea

    D. Shallow respirations

200. Mr. G. has intermittent periods of confusion and cannot report his pain on 0-10 number scale. In order to manage his pain, the best alternative is to

    A. Ask family members to characterize Mr. G.'s pain

    B. Check for changes in vital signs as indicators of pain

    C. Maintain the current long-acting pain medication dose

    D. Try an alternate pain scale

201. In supporting family members at the time of death it is important to

    A. Maintain a continual nursing presence

    B. Encourage family members to leave the body as soon as possible

    C. Ask family members when they want privacy

    D. Ensure that prayers are said at the bedside

198. Answer is B

   A. Incorrect: Patients without formal religious beliefs or practices may still entertain spiritual questions at the end of life.

   B. **Correct**: "Why" questions are part of the search for meaning at the end of life.

   C. Incorrect: Spiritual issues are part of end of life regardless of control.

   D. Incorrect: Patients may prefer to discuss spiritual issues with family members or members of the hospice/palliative team.

199. Answer is A

   A. **Correct**: Dyspnea is the patient's experience of breathlessness and can be quite distressing even when mild.

   B. Incorrect: A Cheyne-Stokes breathing pattern usually occurs after a patient has lost consciousness and is more distressing to family members than the patient.

   C. Incorrect: Periods of apnea are not necessarily distressing to the patient.

   D. Incorrect: Shallow respirations are not necessarily uncomfortable for the patient.

200. Answer is D

   A. Incorrect: This would be a step later—once Mr. G.'s confusion is continuous.

   B. Incorrect: Vital signs are not a reliable indicator in chronic pain.

   C. Incorrect: Interventions should not be maintained at the current level unless reassessment occurs periodically.

   D. **Correct**: An alternate pain scale may be easier for Mr. G. to use even when he is slightly confused.

201. Answer is C

   A. Incorrect: Continual nursing presence may not be needed for patient care or welcomed by the family.

   B. Incorrect: Family members should take the time needed to say their good-byes.

   C. **Correct**: Assessing family members' desires is important in meeting needs.

   D. Incorrect: Prayers are appropriate when patients and/or family members request this specific intervention.

202. Which would be the most appropriate quality indicator for measuring family grief support?

   A. Feeling prepared for loved one's death

   B. Length of grieving period

   C. Frequency of grief counseling

   D. Availability of grief support resources after death

203. The nurse's 68-year-old patient is in the last hours of life after a lengthy illness. The patient has been receiving opioids for pain management. In assessing the patient as death approaches, the nurse knows that the opioid dose may need to be

   A. Increased or decreased to maintain pain control

   B. Given only if requested by the patient

   C. Adjusted since neuropathic pain increases as death approaches

   D. Discontinued due to diminished consciousness and altered mental state

204. The nurse is caring for a patient who is very close to death. Of the following assessment findings, which is the most reliable sign of death?

   A. Cheyne-Stokes respirations

   B. Mottling of extremities

   C. Absence of urine output

   D. Fixed, dilated pupils

205. The nurse is caring for an 85-year-old man who is dying. He has been comatose for several days. His respirations are now shallow and rattling. His adult children at the bedside state, "We don't want our father to suffocate." Which action should the nurse take?

   A. Use a suction machine to remove secretions from the mouth and the throat

   B. Sit the patient up and percuss the back to facilitate loosening of congestion

   C. Reassure the family that the rattling is normal and is not causing suffering

   D. Request an order for humidified oxygen to decrease the client's air hunger

202.   Answer is D

  A. Incorrect: Preparation for the death does not measure grief support after the death.

  B. Incorrect: The length of the grieving period does not necessarily indicate adequate or inadequate grief support.

  C. Incorrect: The frequency of grief counseling does not necessarily indicate adequacy of support.

  D. **Correct**: The availability of services indicates that families can obtain grief support as needed/ desired.

203.   Answer is A

  A. **Correct**: Assessment of pain continues in the last hours of life and medication is adjusted according to that assessment.

  B. Incorrect: If you wait until the patient requests medication, the pain may become out of control.

  C. Incorrect: Neuropathic pain does not necessarily increase as death approaches.

  D. Incorrect: Medication may be reduced if there is reduced renal or hepatic clearance, but otherwise if the patient has been in pain prior to the last few hours, the regimen should be continued. The route of administration may need to be changed if the patient cannot swallow due to the decreased level of consciousness.

204.   Answer is D

  A. Incorrect: Continued respirations are incompatible with death.

  B. Incorrect: Mottling can occur before death.

  C. Incorrect: Absence of urine output may occur before death.

  D. **Correct**: Fixed, dilated pupils are a reliable sign of death.

205.   Answer is C

  A. Incorrect: Shallow, rattling respirations are not an indication for oropharyngeal suctioning.

  B. Incorrect: Congestion at this stage may be interstitial and percussion will not assist in clearing the rattle.

  C. **Correct**: Validating normal signs/symptoms of death and dying and that the patient is comfortable are important nursing interventions at the end of life.

  D. Incorrect: There is no indication from the case description that the patient is experiencing air hunger.

206. The nurse is caring for a woman in a long-term care facility who has a diagnosis of metastatic uterine cancer. She is in the dying process when she suddenly opens her eyes and urgently states, "I need to go . . . I must go now!" Which of the following actions should the nurse take first?

    A. Assess the patency of the woman's urinary catheter and explain that the catheter will take care of her need to urinate

    B. Reorient the woman, reminding her that she is now living in the long-term care facility and that she is safe

    C. Remind the woman who you are and ask her where she needs to go, recognizing she may be exhibiting nearing death awareness

    D. Provide touch and reassurance, recognizing that the woman is most likely confused and agitated due to dehydration

207. The nurse is caring for a man who is imminently dying. During morning care, the man asks the nurse if he is dying. An example of the best response for the nurse to give is

    A. "Yes. Tell me about any concerns, fears, or questions you have about what will happen."

    B. "Yes. I suppose you've known this all along. I promise I'll be right with you all the way."

    C. "Not today. Why don't we look at some of the things you would like to accomplish now?"

    D. "Why do you ask that? You look so much better today than you did yesterday!"

208. The nurse is caring for a patient who is approaching death. Which of the following is the most common sign of imminent death?

    A. Decrease in the swallow reflex

    B. Change in breathing pattern

    C. Weakness and fatigue

    D. Dyspnea

206. Answer is C

   A. Incorrect: In this situation, the patient's expressions are more indicative of a psychological or spiritual need than a physical one and should direct the nurse's first action.

   B. Incorrect: The nurse may lose an opportunity to explore the patient's concerns by emphasizing basic realities.

   C. **Correct**: The nurse is responding with a reminder of her presence so that the patient knows she is not alone and begins exploring her desires further to validate whether this could be an expression of nearing death awareness.

   D. Incorrect: While these actions are not incompatible with therapeutic intervention, this is not the best answer in responding to the patient's specific expression of need.

207. Answer is A

   A. **Correct**: The nurse responds affirmatively but also gives the patient an opportunity to discuss in further detail.

   B. Incorrect: The nurse is responding as if the patient asked a literal question about whether he was dying this instant and loses the opportunity to explore this topic with the patient further.

   C. Incorrect: The nurse should not give false reassurance because she cannot be available 24/7.

   D. Incorrect: This response shuts down dialogue about this important topic.

208. Answer is B

   A. Incorrect: A decrease in the swallowing reflex is not a common, observable sign of imminent death.

   B. **Correct**: Breathing pattern changes are common and may be disconcerting to family members and so it is important to teach them about what to expect.

   C. Incorrect: Weakness and fatigue are not specific to imminent death and occur much earlier and more frequently in the course of illness.

   D. Incorrect: Dyspnea is not specific to imminent death and may occur much earlier in the course of illness.

209. Death "rattle" can be decreased by administering

    A. Sympathomimetics

    B. Aminoglycosides

    C. Anticholinergics

    D. Vasodilators

210. Dehydration is very common in the terminal phases of illness. Which of these statements is true about dehydration in the hospice patient? Dehydration is

    A. Often treated because the patient will be more comfortable

    B. Never treated because it has advantages in the dying patient

    C. Considered a medical emergency and is always treated

    D. Considered a natural part of the dying process and it is most often not necessary to treat

211. Which of the following is the most common symptom associated with patients experiencing dehydration at the end of life?

    A. Abdominal cramps

    B. Nausea

    C. Thirst

    D. Dry mouth

209. Answer is C

   A. Incorrect: Sympathomimetics cause vasoconstriction and therefore would not decrease secretions.

   B. Incorrect: Aminoglycosides are anti-infective agents and would not decrease secretions.

   C. **Correct**: Anticholinergic agents have antisecretory properties. These agents should be given at the first sign of moisture because they will not dry up secretions already present. Agents include scopolamine and hyoscyamine.

   D. Incorrect: Vasodilators act on the blood vessels and would not decrease secretions.

210. Answer is D

   A. Incorrect: Dehydration is truly considered a natural part of the dying process. To treat it would cause more discomfort due to ascites, nausea/vomiting, congestion, and the need to urinate more frequently.

   B. Incorrect: We cannot arbitrarily state that dehydration is never treated. Patient comfort and patient/family wishes are part of the decision process.

   C. Incorrect: Dehydration is not a medical emergency at the end of life.

   D. **Correct**: Dehydration is considered a part of the dying process. Not treating dehydration can decrease cough and congestion, edema and ascites, nausea and vomiting and will decrease the frequency of urination, which can actually improve the quality of life.

211. Answer is D

   A. Incorrect: Abdominal cramps are a sign of acute dehydration in an otherwise healthy individual.

   B. Incorrect: Nausea is not a symptom of dehydration.

   C. Incorrect: Patients at the end of life do not commonly experience thirst due to dehydration.

   D. **Correct**: Dry mouth is a common symptom at the end of life and should be managed with comfort measures.

212. The nurse is caring for a patient who has just died. In caring for the body after death, the goal of care is to

A. Make sure the body is sent to the morgue within an hour after death

B. Have the family members participate in the bathing and dressing the deceased

C. Notify all family members and team members regarding the patient's death

D. Provide a clean, peaceful impression of the deceased for the family

213. The nurse is caring for a patient who has just died. The family is weeping at the bedside. In assisting the family to understand what will occur next, the nurse should

A. Explain how the body will be cared for immediately following the death

B. Request that the family leave the room in order for the body to be washed

C. Give information about the need to remove the body promptly for embalming

D. Ask if they would like to have all the tubes, catheters, and IV lines removed

214. The nurse may experience feelings of anxiety and grief when caring for clients and families facing death and the dying process. In order for the nurse to be able to continue to provide quality care, it is important to obtain personal support by

A. Maintaining an emotional distance from clients and families

B. Periodic transfer to another unit to avoid caring for dying patients

C. Seeking out the assistance of team members whenever necessary

D. Scheduling counseling at regular intervals to deal with loss issues

212. Answer is D

    A. Incorrect: The body should be prepared and family members should be given an opportunity to say good-bye prior to removal if desired. A short time frame isn't required.

    B. Incorrect: This is not a goal of care although it may be provided if family requests.

    C. Incorrect: The family will normally contact other members not present unless they request the nurse to do so.

    D. **Correct**: This is the primary goal of caring for the body after death so that the family can have the best impression before the body is removed to the morgue or funeral home.

213. Answer is A

    A. **Correct**: By providing information the nurse can assist the family in taking the initial steps in grieving and closure for the death event.

    B. Incorrect: Options should always be given to family members instead of directions.

    C. Incorrect: This is not a requirement.

    D. Incorrect: Protocol needs to be followed in removing medical devices.

214. Answer is C

    A. Incorrect: Maintaining emotional distance from clients and families is not appropriate in maintaining a therapeutic and caring relationship.

    B. Incorrect: Avoidance does not promote healthy coping with feelings of anxiety and grief.

    C. **Correct**: The interdisciplinary team is a source of support and guidance for the individual members.

    D. Incorrect: While counseling may be beneficial at specific points, it is not required for a professional to schedule counseling at regular intervals to address loss issues.

Future Trends

215. Which of the following statements is correct concerning healthcare delivery in the future?

    A. The nursing shortage will peak in the year 2010 and then is expected to decline

    B. The number of people with Alzheimer's disease will more than triple from 2001 to 2020

    C. The average life expectancy will be 74 years for males and 79 years for females

    D. The Medicare Trust will be bankrupt by 2010

216. Which of the following best describes advanced care planning and advanced directives?

    A. Can be a serious detriment to communication of end-of-life preferences

    B. Can facilitate greater access to palliative care and hospice services

    C. Must be completed by the patient's primary care physician

    D. Can be activated only when there is no proxy decision-maker

217. Which of the following best describes major barriers to hospice care?

    A. The six-month prognostic requirement results in delayed referral and access to hospice

    B. The Medicare Modernization Act passed by Congress in 2003 revamped the Hospice Medicare Benefit to eliminate barriers to care

    C. The development of palliative care programs in hospitals and nursing homes nationwide has reduced the need for hospice care

    D. Barriers to hospice care remain in rural areas but are not a problem in major cities

215. Answer is B

    A. Incorrect: The nursing shortage will continue without declining beyond 2006.

    B. **Correct**: The number of people with Alzheimer's disease will increase from 4 million to 14 million during this time period.

    C. Incorrect: This is the current life expectancy but it will most likely continue to increase.

    D. Incorrect: The government has predicted bankruptcy by 2020, but there is no definite year that it will happen.

216. Answer is B

    A. Incorrect: Discussion and communication about preferences is beneficial.

    B. **Correct**: Clarity of goals of care can facilitate access to services.

    C. Incorrect: Advance directives are completed by the patient.

    D. Incorrect: Guide care of all decision-makers.

217. Answer is A

    A. **Correct**: The six-month prognosis certification requirement is a major barrier to hospice care.

    B. Incorrect: The Medicare Modernization Act did not significantly revamp the Hospice Medicare Benefit.

    C. Incorrect: The development of palliative care programs may increase access to hospice care services.

    D. Incorrect: Barriers to hospice care remain in both rural and urban areas.

218. Which of the following best describes the potential for reform in end-of-life care?

   A. Success of end-of-life care reform is best accomplished when left to policymakers with the ability to impact legislation

   B. Reform of quality end-of-life care is unlikely over the next two decades given the financial constraints of the healthcare system

   C. Successful reform will involve partnership at every level including provider organizations, public interest groups, government, healthcare professionals, advocacy groups, and others

   D. Hospice and palliative care programs currently provide comprehensive, quality care and there is no need for reform

219. Over the next decade of hospice and palliative care, the primary role of nursing will most likely include

   A. Providing skilled assessment, supportive interventions, consumer education, care coordination, and program leadership

   B. Developing prognostic criteria for the timely referral of patients to hospice and palliative care

   C. Researching models of care to meet the end-of-life needs of an aging population

   D. Promoting healthcare reform to cover the uninsured at end-of-life

220. Which of the following is the most accurate description of the role of unlicensed personnel in palliative care?

   A. Provide emotional support and counseling for family caregivers

   B. Provide physical care to assist in activities of daily living, personal care, and promotion of quality of life

   C. Assist with medication administration and assessing status changes when a nurse is not available

   D. Do not have a significant role in palliative care due to the complexity and severity of illness at the end of life

218. Answer is C

    A. Incorrect: Reform requires the involvement of multiple parties.

    B. Incorrect: Financial constraints exist but this does not necessarily mean that reform is unlikely as reform may decrease healthcare costs.

    C. **Correct**: Reform is most likely to be successful with the involvement of multiple stakeholders.

    D. Incorrect: There is room for improvement in the provision of hospice and palliative care services.

219. Answer is A

    A. **Correct**: All of these components are important aspects of the nursing role in hospice and palliative care.

    B. Incorrect: Developing prognostic criteria is generally outside of the scope of nursing practice.

    C. Incorrect: Researching models of care is not a primary role of nursing.

    D. Incorrect: Though important, promoting coverage for the uninsured is not a primary role of palliative care nursing.

220. Answer is B

    A. Incorrect: Counseling is beyond the scope of unlicensed personnel.

    B. **Correct**: Unlicensed personnel assist with a variety of activities to promote quality of life.

    C. Incorrect: Medication administration and assessment is beyond the scope of practice for unlicensed personnel.

    D. Incorrect: Unlicensed personnel have a very significant role to play in providing care, especially in home and long term care settings.

221. The National Consensus Project for Quality Palliative Care released Clinical Practice Guidelines for Palliative Care in 2004. Which of the following best describes these guidelines?

    A. Can be used as a framework to encourage the development of quality palliative care clinical programs, education, and research.

    B. Includes specific protocols and algorithms for the provision of palliative care services.

    C. Intended as a guideline for appropriate utilization of palliative care services.

    D. Developed to guide the appropriate reimbursement of palliative care services.

222. Which of the following is the best description of trends in the United States that will impact the future of hospice and palliative care?

    A. The increasing federal budget deficit will require a major reduction in the reimbursement of hospice and palliative care over the next decade

    B. Hospice programs will be eliminated, as palliative care becomes the predominant delivery model for end-of-life care

    C. In an effort to further reduce end-of-life care costs, the interdisciplinary care model will be replaced by a primary nursing model

    D. Numerous public health issues including increasing chronic disease, the aging population, health cost containment and other factors mean that the demand for quality palliative care will increase significantly

223. The groundbreaking SUPPORT study, funded by the Robert Wood Johnson Foundation and published in the Journal of the American Medical Association in 1995 revealed the following

    A. Support personnel in healthcare provide the majority of end-of-life care

    B. Findings of serious deficiencies in end-of-life care, use of advance directives, and relief of pain

    C. Patients and families are overburdened economically and emotionally in providing end-of-life care in the home

    D. Healthcare professionals need support in providing quality end-of-life care

221. Answer is A

    A. **Correct**: This is the stated purpose of these guidelines.

    B. Incorrect: The guidelines provide standards for clinical practice and care but not specific protocols for pain or symptom management.

    C. Incorrect: The guidelines are not a utilization review document.

    D. Incorrect: The guidelines do not provide reimbursement criteria for palliative care services.

222. Answer is D

    A. Incorrect: The federal budget deficit is increasing but will not necessarily require a reduction in reimbursement for palliative care.

    B. Incorrect: There is no prediction that hospice care will be eliminated.

    C. Incorrect: There is no prediction that interdisciplinary care will be eliminated.

    D. **Correct**: Demand (need) for services will definitely increase.

223. Answer is B

    A. Incorrect: Support personnel do provide significant care at the end-of-life but this was not a finding of the study.

    B. **Correct**: This was the major conclusion of the study.

    C. Incorrect: The study did not focus on the experience of patients and families in home care.

    D. Incorrect: While a solution to some of the findings of the study might be more support through training and education of healthcare professionals in end-of-life care, this was not a finding of the study.

224. Hospice nurses can promote the use of the Clinical Practice Guidelines for Quality Palliative Care developed by the National Consensus Project in all of the following ways **EXCEPT**

A. Suggest an in-service training program to introduce the staff to the guidelines

B. Compare and contrast the hospice agency's existing guidelines with the Clinical Practice Guidelines and note areas of consistency or divergence

C. Request an immediate change in the agency model of care when discrepancies are found with the national standards

D. Participate in ongoing quality improvement activities to assess potential effectiveness of national standards within an agency

Advanced Care Planning

225. Which approach by the nurse is most appropriate in caring for a dying patient?

A. Assist the patient and family to make choices regarding the final stage of life

B. Explore choices that will avoid suffering for the patient and family

C. Make decisions about physical care for the family to reduce their stress

D. Advocate for the family to complete an advance directive for the patient

226. While caring for a woman with advanced multiple sclerosis, the hospice nurse is discussing advance directives with her. Which statement by the patient indicates understanding of advance directives?

A. "I need to ask my attorney to prepare the advance directive."

B. "I can't change my healthcare proxy once the document is signed."

C. "I can revise my end-of-life options in the advance directives."

D. "I must also complete a living will when I'm admitted to a hospital."

224. Answer is C

    A. Incorrect: This would be an appropriate step to take to increase awareness of the guidelines and engage staff in dialogue about the guidelines.

    B. Incorrect: This would be a worthwhile analysis before initiating any changes in practice, policy or procedure.

    C. **Correct**: Immediate changes without analysis, discussion and planning would be inappropriate. There may be valid rationale that supports deviation from the standards in a particular setting or agency.

    D. Incorrect: This would be another worthwhile activity to validate the standards in actual practice.

Advanced Care Planning

225. Answer is A

    A. **Correct**: The nurse has information and resources she can provide to the patient and family in assisting them to make choices consistent with their values, needs, and preferences.

    B. Incorrect: The patient and family determine the goals of the care and the nurse can assist with appropriate choices.

    C. Incorrect: The patient and family should be involved in decision-making about care.

    D. Incorrect: The patient should be able to make his/her own advance directive.

226. Answer is C

    A. Incorrect: The patient does not need an attorney to prepare an advance directive.

    B. Incorrect: A healthcare proxy can most definitely be changed by the patient at a later point if desired.

    C. **Correct**: The patient can revise end-of-life options in the advance directives if desired.

    D. Incorrect: There is no requirement for living will completion. Patients are encouraged to consider advance directives when they are admitted.

227. In palliative care, the nurse cares for patients for whom life-saving techniques may no longer be appropriate. Which statement about "Do Not Resuscitate" (DNR) status is true?

   A. Is usually is a legal requirement for admission to a hospice program

   B. Requires a written physician's order in the patient's record

   C. Is not applicable outside of the hospital or emergency room setting

   D. Includes stopping life-sustaining treatment such as a ventilator

228. The nurse is caring for a client in the end stages of a long illness. When determining the benefit of treatment or therapy with the patient and family, which question is the **LEAST** important to consider? Does the

   A. Treatment or therapy match the patient/family goals of care

   B. Benefit of treatment or therapy outweigh the risks

   C. Treatment or therapy ensure comfort and quality life closure

   D. Treatment or therapy prolong the life of the patient

229. Mr. Smith is hospitalized with a brain tumor. He is intermittently confused. He has completed a Living Will stating his wishes to have no extraordinary measures. His brother disagrees and requests that "everything possible" be done to prolong Mr. Smith's life. The patient's wishes should be

   A. Ignored because the family member disagrees

   B. Respected as written in the living will

   C. Discussed with family members and respected

   D. Aggressive care should be immediately started

227. Answer is B

    A. Incorrect: DNR is not a legal requirement for admission to a hospice program although patients are informed of the hospice philosophy of care and are provided informed consent for the Hospice Medicare Benefit.

    B. **Correct**: DNR status either in the hospital or out of the hospital requires a physician's order.

    C. Incorrect: DNR is applicable outside of the hospital; it is called a non-hospital DNR.

    D. Incorrect: DNR status would mean that patients would not receive further cardio-pulmonary resuscitation but does not necessarily require that a ventilator be removed.

228. Answer is D

    A. Incorrect: This is the most important consideration.

    B. Incorrect: Considering the benefits and burdens of proposed therapies is very important in determining priorities at the end of life.

    C. Incorrect: Comfort and closure are usually important goals for patients at the end of life.

    D. **Correct**: Prolongation of life is not usually a primary consideration at the end of life.

229. Answer is C

    A. Incorrect: Healthcare workers have an obligation to honor the patient's wishes as written in the Living Will.

    B. Incorrect: The Living Will must be respected but a discussion needs to also occur with the family members to assist and support their concerns while educating about the patient's wishes.

    C. **Correct**: Since the Living Will was completed when the patient was competent, it must be respected. Discussing these issues with family members helps the brother recognize these were the wishes of the patient.

    D. Incorrect: Aggressive care would be totally inappropriate in this situation.

230. The patient lacks decision-making capacity and has no Durable Power of Attorney for Healthcare. He is appropriate for hospice. Which of the following persons could **NOT**, under any circumstances, legally sign the consent?

    A. A non-related employee of the hospice

    B. A next-door neighbor who has known the patient for over 20 years

    C. His wife

    D. His attorney

231. Mr. L is a 78-year-old mildly demented male admitted to hospice post motor vehicle accident with head trauma and internal bleeding. Mr. L's wife died as a result of the accident. Mr. L has only one living son. Mr. L appears intermittently confused. What should be examined in order to develop a plan of care?

    A. Had Mr. L's wife shown signs of caregiver fatigue prior to the accident

    B. His decision-making capacity needs to be determined

    C. Did Mr. L have a living will or advance directive

    D. What are the son's wishes about Mr. L's care

232. Which of the following statements about ethics is true?

    A. Ethics are the social customs, norms and rules that define "right" and "wrong"

    B. Ethics are not influenced by culture

    C. Nurses should be guided only by their personal morals

    D. Ethics change over time

230. Answer is A

    A. **Correct**: The non-related employee is an illegal representative and could not under any circumstance, legally sign the consent.

    B. Incorrect: The individual would be legal if the patient named this person as a surrogate decision maker.

    C. Incorrect: The wife is the next of kin and therefore is the first to be considered for legal decision-making.

    D. Incorrect: The attorney could be a surrogate decision maker if named by the patient.

231. Answer is B

    A. Incorrect: Decision-making is the main concern to move forward with Mr. L's plan of care.

    B. **Correct**: His decision-making capacity needs to be determined. If Mr. L were deemed to be able to make decisions, he would speak for himself. If not, his healthcare proxy or advanced directive would be used to direct care according to his wishes.

    C. Incorrect: Decision-making capacity is the primary concern but all documents should be examined that indicate the patient's preferences.

    D. Incorrect: Although the son is the next of kin, the patient's wishes must be honored if these are known. Otherwise, the son would be advised to make decisions for the father with his best interest in mind.

232. Answer is D

    A. Incorrect: Morals are the social customs, norms, and rules that define right and wrong. Ethics are methods used to understand and examine the moral life. Ethics is also a branch of philosophy that focuses on the moral life.

    B. Incorrect: Ethics are influenced by culture.

    C. Incorrect: Although nurses are influenced by their personal morals and should not have to act against those morals, they should understand the ethical principles and concepts that influence healthcare and nursing care. They also should be knowledgeable about the laws that govern nursing care and the ethical positions of professional nursing organizations.

    D. **Correct**: Ethics are not immutable because they occur in an ever-changing socio-cultural context.

233. The bioethical principle that forms the basis of informed consent is

   A. Futility

   B. Nonmaleficence

   C. Autonomy

   D. Justice

234. The process of resolving ethical dilemmas

   A. Is similar to the nursing process

   B. Relies completely on discussing the medical facts of the case

   C. Always results in the right answer if procedures are followed carefully

   D. Requires input from lawyers

235. The nurse is caring for a 10-year-old girl in the terminal stages of cancer. The child has not been eating for the past 3 days. During a family meeting, the parents state that they are concerned about her "starving to death" and ask if they should agree to have a feeding tube placed. All of the following interventions are appropriate actions for the nurse to take **EXCEPT**

   A. Explain the benefits of dehydration during the dying process

   B. Discuss the family's concerns about feeding or not feeding the child

   C. Assess the child's symptoms—including hunger, thirst and dry mouth—and instruct the family on ways to provide comfort care

   D. Contact the physician to have a feeding tube placed

233. Answer is C

A. Incorrect: Futility is the determination that a therapy will not benefit a patient and therefore should not be prescribed. Futility may influence a person's choice about a particular therapy but futility is not always involved in informed consent.

B. Incorrect: Nonmaleficence is the obligation of a clinician to avoid harming the patient or exposing the patient to unnecessary risks. This principle often is invoked when discussing treatments with patients and families that may cause more suffering without maintaining or increasing the patient's quality of life. It is one consideration for informed consent but is not the key principle underlying informed consent.

C. **Correct**: Autonomy is the individual's right to choose freely. Informed consent depends on a person being able to exercise his choice.

D. Incorrect: Justice involves the fair and equitable treatment of patients and their families. The issue of justice usually focuses on the allocation of healthcare resources rather than informed consent.

234. Answer is A

A. **Correct**: Resolving ethical dilemmas should use a problem-solving approach. The nursing process is an example of a problem-solving approach.

B. Incorrect: Resolving ethical dilemmas includes clinical information but must also incorporate information about the patient's and family's values and goals, identification of key decision makers and consideration of the ethical principles that influence the situation.

C. Incorrect: Ethical issues do not have clear "right" or "wrong" answers. Resolving ethical dilemmas means that one makes the best choice based on the information considered in answer "B."

D. Incorrect: Most ethical dilemmas can be resolved without input from the legal system.

235. Answer is D

A. Incorrect: This is an appropriate action

B. Incorrect: See A

C. Incorrect: See A

D. **Correct**: This is not an appropriate action for the nurse to take until the family has explored options, been provided with information and had the opportunity to make an informed decision.

236. In the context of irreversible illness, withholding and withdrawing life-sustaining therapies

    A. Are generally accepted as ethical acts

    B. Do not include tube feedings

    C. May be referred to as "mercy killing"

    D. Are also called active euthanasia

237. Which of the following statements about administering opioids to dying patients is true?

    A. Administering opioids to treat pain in dying patients is an act of euthanasia

    B. Administering opioid therapy if there is a risk of hastening death is never ethically and legally justified

    C. There is research indicating that administering opioids at the end of life does not hasten death

    D. Nurses have no obligation to provide opioids to dying patients in pain if they think that this will hasten death

238. Euthanasia is

    A. Widely accepted as an ethical practice

    B. Currently legal only in Oregon State

    C. Defended as a practice that upholds the sanctity of life

    D. Different from assisted suicide

236. Answer is A

    A. **Correct**: Withholding and withdrawing life-sustaining therapies are widely accepted in state laws, court decisions and by bioethicists, professional healthcare organizations, and most religious traditions.

    B. Incorrect: Tube feedings are considered medical therapies that can be refused by patients.

    C. Incorrect: Mercy killing is a term applied to euthanasia.

    D. Incorrect: Active euthanasia is acting to end the life of a patient to relieve the patient's suffering. This usually involves administration of a lethal injection.

237. Answer is C

    A. Incorrect: A is a false statement because euthanasia is the act of putting to death a person to relieve the person's suffering. In euthanasia, the intent is to end someone's life, whereas the intent of administering opioids is to relieve pain rather than ending the person's life.

    B. Incorrect: B is a false statement. The Rule of Double Effect (RDE) provides ethical justification for actions that have positive intended effects (e.g., relieving pain) and negative unintended but foreseen (e.g., hastening death) effects.

    C. **Correct**: C is a true statement. Several studies have found no evidence that administering opioids shortens a person's life.

    D. Incorrect: D is a false statement. Several organizations, including the Hospice and Palliative Nurses Association and the American Nurses Association, have published statements that emphasize the moral obligation that nurses have to relieve pain in dying patients.

238. Answer is D

    A. Incorrect: Although there is much debate about whether or not assisted death (which includes both euthanasia and assisted suicide) is ethical, assisted death is not widely accepted as being ethical.

    B. Incorrect: Assisted suicide is legal in Oregon but euthanasia is not. Currently, euthanasia is illegal everywhere in the United States.

    C. Incorrect: An argument against euthanasia and assisted suicide contends that these practices violate the sanctity of life.

    D. **Correct**: In euthanasia, another person (usually a physician) acts to end the life of a patient to relieve the patient's suffering. In assisted suicide, the clinician provides the means (usually a lethal dose of barbiturates) for the patient to end his own life.

239. Which of the following statements accurately reflects ways in which culture affects ethical decision-making?

    A. Culture does not affect the way people make ethical decisions

    B. Some cultures believe that telling the patient that they have a terminal illness is disrespectful and/or injurious

    C. In general, patient autonomy is the highest value that guides decision-makers from traditional cultures

    D. Although people from non-European American cultures often have different values that guide ethical decisions, nurses are legally bound to follow the values of the American healthcare system

240. Conscientious objection is

    A. Illegal in the United States

    B. Permitted if the nurse obtains permission from his/her state board of nursing not to participate in a patient's care

    C. Permitted if the nurse lacks the knowledge to care for the patient

    D. Acceptable as long as the patient's and family's wishes are respected

239.   Answer is B

    A. Incorrect: Culture greatly influences how people make ethical decisions.

    B. **Correct**: Some cultures do not value truth telling because they believe that it shows disrespect to the patient and can also be a great burden to the patient, causing the patient to lose hope.

    C. Incorrect: Traditional cultures tend to emphasize the role of the family and the community in caring for the patient and in making decisions.

    D. Incorrect: Nurses and other healthcare providers must practice within legal boundaries. They should strive to respect patients' and families' values. However, if the patient does not want the information or requests that the information be given to family members, then that wish should be documented in the chart and honored.

240.   Answer is D

    A. Incorrect: Conscientious objection or the right of persons to refuse to participate in acts that they deem unethical, is widely accepted in healthcare practice today. It allows clinicians who are morally opposed to such acts as abortion, capital punishment, and assisted suicide to abstain from caring for patients in these circumstances.

    B. Incorrect: Nurses do not need special permission from any official body. However, they must assure that the patient is not abandoned and his wishes are honored.

    C. Incorrect: Lack of knowledge is not an acceptable reason to object to caring for a patient. The nurse must object to caring for the patient on moral grounds.

    D. **Correct**: The patient and family must receive the care and not be abandoned.

241. Which statement accurately reflects the relationship between the concepts of legality and ethics?

   A. There is no relationship between what is legal and what is ethical

   B. Legal actions are always ethical

   C. Ethical actions can be illegal

   D. The U.S. Supreme Court determines if an action is ethical or not

242. Mrs. Nguyen is a patient with advanced dementia who is unresponsive and completely dependent for her physical needs. Her son asks the team to advise him about whether or not to agree to the placement of a percutaneous gastrostomy tube for enteral feeding. What bioethical concept is most likely to influence the conversation?

   A. Justice

   B. Futility

   C. Rule of Double Effect

   D. Beneficence

243. An 84-year-old widow with diabetes and end-stage renal disease has been sent to the hospital from a nursing home. She has gangrene of the left foot with multiple, open infected wounds. Surgery is recommended, but the client does not want any invasive procedures. She wants to go back to the nursing home. She is alert, oriented and has good decision-making capacity. Her children are emotionally distraught and pull the nurse aside to say, "We want the surgery. We want to do everything that can be done." What should the nurse do first?

   A. Ensure the client and family understand the treatment options and risks

   B. Ask the hospital ethics committee to consider this case as soon as possible

   C. Offer to discuss the children's preferences with the physicians

   D. Encourage the children to talk their mother into having the surgery

241.   Answer is C

    A.   Incorrect: Laws are guided by societal ethics.

    B.   Incorrect: Many legal actions are considered unethical by some people; examples include assisted suicide (in Oregon and Washington States), abortion and capital punishment.

    C.   **Correct**: Some actions, such as civil disobedience, are considered ethical but not legal. Some people believe that certain illegal acts such as euthanasia are ethical.

    D.   Incorrect: The U.S. Supreme Court decides whether or not a situation or act is constitutional. Although the U.S. Constitution and its interpretation are based on values and ethics, the court does not decide a case based on these criteria.

242.   Answer is B

    A.   Incorrect: Justice refers to treating people fairly. Justice should not be a factor in this decision.

    B.   **Correct**: Placing a feeding tube is unlikely to enhance Ms. Nguyen's quality of life, but may result in several complications, such as bleeding, infection, and fluid overload. Because this treatment is unlikely to help the patient and may harm her, the team will advise her son that the therapy is medically futile.

    C.   Incorrect: The Rule of Double Effect justifies an action that can have both good and bad outcomes. Tube feeding is unlikely to have any good outcomes and thus is not justified.

    D.   Incorrect: Although the team has an obligation to help Mrs. Nguyen, that is "to do good," this principle is not the major one guiding this decision.

243.   Answer is A

    A.   **Correct**: Informed consent is the principle underlying this action.

    B.   Incorrect: The first action is for the nurse to assess client/family understanding and provide information. If a conflict still exists, then an ethics consult would be warranted.

    C.   Incorrect: The patient still has decision-making capacity.

    D.   Incorrect: Encouraging the children to discuss the matter with their mother would be appropriate nursing action, but not encouraging them to persuade her.

244. The nurse is caring for a middle-aged man with end stage amyotrophic lateral sclerosis (ALS). The man's son and daughter have cared for him for the past 2 years and now he is physically dependent on them. The patient has just broached the subject of assisted suicide with the nurse and says he plans to discuss the subject with his children that evening. The nurse's first response should be to

A. Notify the physician and the nurse manager so that appropriate measures can be implemented

B. Offer to discuss the patient's preference with the family so that they are not surprised by the idea

C. Respect the patient's confidentiality by waiting for the family to discuss the issue first

D. Recognize that the patient may have unmet end-of-life needs that require prompt assessment

245. The nurse is caring for a client with end-stage chronic obstructive pulmonary disease (COPD) who is dying. The client's respirations are labored with frequent episodes of apnea and restlessness. The nurse administers the prescribed morphine for comfort and shortness of breath. The client dies 20 minutes later. Which ethical principles best support the nurse's action?

A. Veracity and autonomy

B. Beneficence and double effect

C. Patient self-determination and justice

D. Nonmaleficence and medical futility

246. The hospice nurse is caring for a dying patient whose family disagrees with the patient's decisions about end-of-life care. Which action should the nurse take first?

A. Present the case to the agency's ethics committee for a resolution

B. Ask the healthcare team to have a conference regarding end-of-life care

C. Initiate a referral to social services and request a home visit

D. Encourage the family and client to discuss the conflict

244. Answer is D

    A. Incorrect: Nursing process indicates that further assessment is the first response.

    B. Incorrect: The nurse can encourage the patient to discuss his thoughts and feelings with his family but it is not appropriate for the nurse to act on his behalf.

    C. Incorrect: The nurse can respect the patient's confidentiality while still exploring the issue further with the patient and making appropriate supportive referrals.

    D. **Correct**: Nursing process indicates that further assessment is the first and best response.

245. Answer is B

    A. Incorrect: Veracity is truth telling and autonomy is the act of choosing freely.

    B. **Correct**: Beneficence, the obligation to do good and double effect, the principle that actions with positive intended effects are ethically justified even if there are negative unintended effects.

    C. Incorrect: The patient is no longer able to make choices freely.

    D. Incorrect: While medical treatment with a curative purpose may be futile at this stage, providing comfort is an obligation.

246. Answer is D

    A. Incorrect: While there is a conflict, this is not the indicated first action.

    B. Incorrect: See A

    C. Incorrect: See A

    D. **Correct**: Once the nurse has assessed the situation and verified the presence of disagreement between patient and family, encouraging and supporting discussion and dialogue is the best first step toward resolution.

247. Ethical issues abound in palliative care. Which statement most accurately describes the nurse's role in addressing ethical issues in palliative care?

    A. Consider patient decisions according to the nurse's own values and beliefs

    B. Help the patient/family understand all options and their potential consequences

    C. Refer patient care ethical issues to ethics experts within the healthcare system

    D. Determine when patients are no longer competent to make their own decisions

248. The nurse is talking with the family of a man who is dying. Which statement by a family member is a correct example of the ethical principle listed?

    A. Confidentiality: "Please don't tell Dad his diagnosis or that he's dying."

    B. Disclosure: "Please don't give Dad's medical information to anyone but me."

    C. Nonmaleficence: "Can we stop the daily weights and lab work since Dad is dying and they cause him pain?"

    D. Competence: "I don't think Dad is able to make decisions for himself so just ask me about any decisions to be made for him and I will."

249. The nurse can contribute to ethical practice in end-of-life care by doing all of the following **EXCEPT**

    A. Work closely with physicians to meet the needs of patients and their families

    B. Ensure that patients/families are aware of treatment options and consequences of those options

    C. Participate in creating systems of care that specifically meet end-of-life needs for patients and families

    D. Use personal values and morals to determine best courses of actions for patients and families

247. Answer is B

    A. Incorrect: Patients should be provided with information and options so that they can make decisions consistent with their own values and beliefs.

    B. **Correct**: In order for patients and families to choose options that fit with their value system they need information about all available options.

    C. Incorrect: Nurses can address ethical issues based on their education and experience. Ethics consults may be requested when dilemmas are difficult to resolve and conflict exists.

    D. Incorrect: In most states physicians are charged with the responsibility for determining a patient's capacity to make decisions.

248. Answer is C

    A. Incorrect: Not telling a patient his diagnosis or that he's dying violates the principle of veracity (truth-telling), not confidentiality.

    B. Incorrect: Disclosure is not an ethical principle.

    C. **Correct**: Nonmaleficence (do not harm) indicates that actions causing the patient pain or discomfort without any benefit should be discontinued.

    D. Incorrect: Competence is not an ethical principle.

249. Answer is D

    A. Incorrect: This is a way that nurses contribute to ethical practice.

    B. Incorrect: See A

    C. Incorrect: See A

    D. **Correct**: This is a false statement. Nurses must work with the preferences and needs of patients and families.

250. The nurse is caring for a man hospitalized with advanced metastatic disease. He has declined further treatment and he is aware that his disease may progress more rapidly. The patient is considered to have good decision-making capacity. Who should make the decision to terminate treatment for this patient and what ethical principle is applicable?

    A. The patient refuses treatment for himself according to the right to self-determination

    B. The physician decides to withdraw treatment based on the principle of medical futility

    C. The family declines further treatment, exerting their option to claim surrogacy or proxy

    D. The executive board determines the patient's competence and applies hospital policies

251. Positive steps to help others or to prevent harm is the definition of

    A. Beneficence

    B. Veracity

    C. Nonmaleficence

    D. Justice

252. Mr. Jones is a 58-year-old male with lung cancer. He has good skin integrity but is in bed most of the time. His family has requested a very expensive specialty bed. What ethical principle would you use to determine if the bed should be provided?

    A. Confidentiality

    B. Autonomy

    C. Beneficence

    D. Justice

253. Truth-telling is the definition of

    A. Justice

    B. Beneficence

    C. Veracity

    D. Fidelity

250. Answer is A

    A. **Correct**: The patient is able to make his own decisions as long as he has capacity. His expressed preferences will continue to be followed if they have been written or communicated to the proxy decision-maker.

    B. Incorrect: While further treatment may be medically futile at this point, the patient should be given the options to make informed decisions while he retains capacity.

    C. Incorrect: Proxy is not active until a patient no longer has capacity.

    D. Incorrect: As long as the patient has capacity, no other authorities have a role in making decisions about his care.

251. Answer is A

    A. **Correct**: This is the definition of beneficence.

    B. Incorrect: Veracity is truth telling.

    C. Incorrect: Nonmaleficence is avoiding the intentional infliction of harm.

    D. Incorrect: Justice is giving others what is due or owed and treating all people fair.

252. Answer is D

    A. Incorrect: Confidentiality is the patient right to maintain privacy regarding personal and medical matters.

    B. Incorrect: Autonomy is an individual's personal liberty.

    C. Incorrect: Beneficence is the duty to help others.

    D. **Correct**: Justice is to consider rules and actions that result in fair and equitable use of available resources.

253. Answer is C

    A. Incorrect: Justice is giving others what is due or owed.

    B. Incorrect: Beneficence is positive steps to help others or to prevent harm.

    C. **Correct**: Truth-telling is the definition of veracity.

    D. Incorrect: Fidelity is establishing trust.

254. The family of an 85-year-old patient with end stage respiratory disease who now lacks decision-making capacity has decided to withdraw treatment consistent with the patient's wishes. Which of the following **CANNOT** be ethically withdrawn by the healthcare team?

A. Antibiotics

B. Ventilator support

C. Cardio-pulmonary resuscitation

D. Comfort care

255. A 75-year-old male patient with end stage prostate cancer is experiencing severe pain, including hyper-algesia/allodynia which is intractable to high doses of opioids and adjuvant analgesics despite the best efforts of the palliative care team. Which of the following is legally and ethically justifiable in the majority of states in the United States?

A. Palliative sedation

B. Assisted suicide

C. Euthanasia

D. Tripling the current dose of opioids

254. Answer is D

   A. Incorrect: Antibiotics can be withdrawn according to the patient's wishes.

   B. Incorrect: Ventilator support can be withdrawn according to the patient and family's wishes regarding life-sustaining therapy.

   C. Incorrect: Patients and families may request a Do Not Resuscitate order.

   D. **Correct**: The team cannot abandon the patient and must continue to provide.

255. Answer is A

   A. **Correct**: Palliative sedation must be considered in cases of intractable pain for relief of suffering.

   B. Incorrect: Assisted suicide is legal only in the state of Oregon and Washington.

   C. Incorrect: Euthanasia is illegal throughout the United States and Canada.

   D. Incorrect: This would not be an effective option since the pain is intractable to high doses; this level of increase suddenly could cause untoward effects.

Case Studies
and Answers

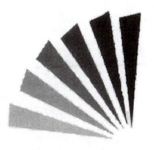

Case Studies for Discussion

Case Study #1

You are caring for a 79-year-old gentleman with advanced prostate cancer with multiple bone metastases. He is taking long-acting morphine and at your visits insists he is doing well even though you have noted a gradual decrease in his activity. For example, he used to spend hours in his woodshop; now he rarely goes there. When you point this out to him, he insists he is "fine."

His daughter, however, has a different story. She reports her dad has severe pain and is not taking all of his scheduled or breakthrough medication because, to use his words, "I don't want to die an addict." She has tried to reassure him by telling him that a person experiencing pain can't become an addict.

1. What additional assessment data should the nurse collect?

2. How should you, the nurse, approach this patient and family about his pain and their concerns regarding opioids for pain control?

3. What information can you provide to both the patient and daughter about addiction?

4. What adjuvant therapy should be considered in this situation?

5. What other actions/interventions are appropriate to implement in this situation?

Case Study #1 Answers

1. **Answer**: The nurse needs to conduct an assessment to explore alternative explanations for the patient's decreased activity including an assessment of other symptoms like nausea, constipation, fatigue, depression, or disease progression. The nurse should also perform a good pain assessment-description of the pain, duration, intensity, location, precipitating, and alleviating factors etc. with special attention to the side effects the patient experiences with the current pain regimen.

2. **Answer**: The nurse needs to explore with the patient and family, the nature of his pain and how it is impacting his quality of life. She can help him see that his pain will change throughout the course of his illness. What is a satisfactory level of pain relief for this patient at this time? What side effects of the medications are most bothersome to the patient and how have they been managed? The nurse also needs to explore the fears regarding addiction in more detail. Has the family had previous experiences with addiction? The nurse can explain the rationale for scheduling medications to prevent pain so that less total medication can be used to keep pain under control.

3. **Answer**: The patient and his daughter can be helped to understand that addiction is not a danger when a person takes opioids for the pain of cancer. The nurse can discuss tolerance versus addiction and also let the patient know that some side effects of the narcotic are transitory.

4. **Answer**: The patient would probably benefit from the addition of a scheduled NSAID, which may further decrease the total needed dose of opioids. Also, has the patient received a radiation therapy consult for possible treatment of affected areas? The patient may also be depressed and that may account for some of the slowdown in his physical activity; if so, the addition of an antidepressant might be indicated. Medications to manage any side effects should be added, most notably stool softeners/laxatives to prevent/treat constipation.

5. **Answer**: The hospice social worker and/or chaplain could visit with the patient to complete a more thorough assessment of any psychosocial and/or spiritual issues that may be affecting the patient and pursue appropriate interventions. The nurse may also offer a volunteer to assist in the woodshop. The nurse should also complete teaching with the patient and family regarding the management of fatigue and expected changes in activity level as the disease progresses.

Case Study #2

You are the on-call nurse and are called to the home of a patient who is experiencing the following signs and symptoms: anxiety, sweating, nausea, vomiting, cramps, and insomnia. You refer to your on-call information and note the patient is on IV morphine at the rate of 5 mg/hour. The patient's wife is concerned that death may be nearing or that her husband is addicted to the morphine.

1. What additional assessment data do you need to gather?

2. What topics may be appropriate to teach the patient and family at this point?

3. What non-pharmacologic approaches are appropriate to implement in this situation?

Case Study #2 Answers

1. **Answer**: These seem to be signs of morphine withdrawal. The nurse needs to gather additional data. What other processes could be causing these symptoms (intestinal obstruction, hypercalcemia)? The nurse needs to know the pain history, as well as the history of the morphine infusion. Has the wife altered the rate out of her fear of the patient's addiction or causing his death? Is the IV functioning properly?

2. **Answer**: It would be helpful for the nurse to probe with the wife about her fears, to explain the signs of impending death and find out if the wife needs additional help. The wife can be helped to understand that addiction is not a valid fear when patients are experiencing pain related to the disease and that the morphine infusion will not hasten the patient's death.

3. **Answer**: The wife and patient need to be reassured that they won't be left "alone" in this situation. It might be helpful to have the nurse phone the home every 6 hours or so for a couple of days to see how things are going. The nurse might explore with the wife whether there are other family members, friends or members of her church that can be present with her at this time. The nurse can offer any additional resources available through the hospice—volunteers, home health aide, etc. If there is a reason to suspect that the wife may be withholding morphine, even after counseling and discussion, the hospice might consider continuous care to monitor the situation or an inpatient hospice admission to ensure the patient's symptoms are adequately assessed and managed.

Case Study #3

Your new patient is a 30-year-old woman with metastatic breast cancer to the hip and spine. She indicates pain in two places: her right hip and mid-thoracic spine. She describes her hip pain as a deep ache, worse when she walks and her back pain as a burning sensation, worse when lying down, that radiates down to her left thigh. Her present medication regimen is oxycodone/acetaminophen 2 tablets every 3 hours around the clock. Her pain scores (on a 0-10 scale) are:

Pain at its best:	hip – 4;	back – 6
Pain at its worst:	hip – 8;	back – 9
Pain now:	hip – 5;	back –7

1. What additional pain assessment information is needed?

2. What type(s) of pain do you think she is experiencing?

3. The physician has asked for your recommendation. How would you change her pain regimen?

4. What non-pharmacological approaches might you try?

Case Study #3 Answers

1. **Answer**: One needs to know how often, in fact, she is taking the oxycodone/acetaminophen combination and how much oxycodone and acetaminophen are in each tablet. The most common combination is 5 mg oxycodone and 325 mg of acetaminophen but the combination can vary with oxycodone 2.5-10 mg and acetaminophen 325-650 mg. How long she has been on this dose; has she had radiation therapy to these areas? Also, what precipitates and alleviates the pain? What other medications is she taking?

2. **Answer**: She is having somatic (bone) pain (described as a deep ache) and neuropathic pain (described as a burning sensation radiating down her left thigh).

3. **Answer**: An NSAID and a tricyclic antidepressant, like nortriptyline should be started to cover bone and neuropathic pain respectively. Oxycodone/acetaminophen should be changed to oxycodone alone and dosed appropriately based on the amount of medication she had been taking, probably 10 mg, but every 4 hours, which is the appropriate dosing interval for oxycodone. Breakthrough dose (10-15% of 24 hour dose given orally every 2 hours as needed) should be 6-9 mg and could be 5-10 mg since this is the dose available in tablets. If this patient had been taking the previous recommended pain regimen she would have been receiving 650 mg of acetaminophen every 3 hours, which equals 5200 mg of acetaminophen or 5.2 Gm, which is significantly greater than the daily maximum dose of 4 Gm. The addition of adjuvant therapies may decrease the need for these doses of opioids but it is important to get the pain controlled and it takes days to weeks before an antidepressant may have significant effect with neuropathic pain. Once pain is controlled, a long acting opioid should be instituted. Sustained release oxycodone would be the preferred choice and if the dose remains the same, would start at 30 mg bid. Stool softeners/laxatives should also be added to the regimen to prevent constipation if they are not already ordered.

4. **Answer**: The patient might benefit from gentle hydrotherapy, as well as planning her ADLs so they are spaced apart and she isn't on her feet for too long at any given time. Attention should be given to positioning in bed and heat and massage might be helpful as well.

Case Study #4

You are caring for a 74-year-old gentleman with end stage COPD and a history of CO_2 retention. Over the weeks you have known him, he has become increasingly short of breath in spite of countless interventions. You feel low-dose morphine, given as needed, is the next logical intervention. The physician is reluctant to give you the order because of concern over respiratory depression. He has never taken opioids before.

1. How might you approach the physician?

2. What starting dose of morphine and route would you recommend?

3. How might the patient's family be assured of morphine's safety?

4. What non-pharmacologic interventions are effective for dyspnea?

5. How might the interdisciplinary team be involved with this patient's care?

Case Study #4 Answers

1. **Answer**: You can talk with the physician and explain that a low dose of oral morphine is used initially to treat dyspnea in opioid naïve patients and that the morphine will be titrated upwards slowly while the patient becomes tolerant to the side effect of respiratory depression. You can also mention the hospice staff's experience with this therapy in similar situations. The hospice staff will also provide appropriate monitoring of respirations and side effects. Family caregivers will also be taught how to appropriately administer the medication and monitor for effects. Also, that morphine is especially effective in treating the air hunger of end stage COPD and that the other interventions have not been effective. Offer to fax a reference or research information on the use of morphine with shortness of breath to the physician.

2. **Answer**: The recommendation would be to start with 5 mg orally every 4 hours PRN, then titrate up as needed and tolerated. Be sure to ask the physician to order a stool softener/laxative and an anti-emetic to control the side effects of the opioid.

3. **Answer**: The family should be assured that morphine is used for shortness of breath frequently and that any side effects will be aggressively managed. They should be reassured that the dose will be carefully titrated upwards if necessary and that addiction is not a concern.

4. **Answer**: The patient might benefit from a fan to circulate air in the room as well as reducing anything in the environment that heightens his sense of being closed in and feeling anxious. Relaxation techniques can also be taught.

5. **Answer**: The social worker and chaplain may be helpful in talking about the special anxiety that comes with shortness of breath, helping to minimize other sources of anxiety and in helping the patient find ways to be calm.

Case Study #5

You are caring for a 60-year-old gentleman with widespread small cell cancer of the lung, metastatic to the bone and liver. He rates his pain as a "10" on a 1-10 scale, especially in his right hip and leg. You note the patient has a 40-year history of heavy alcohol use (about 10 beers a day, plus some bourbon) and has admitted to some marijuana and cocaine use in the past. He reports, at present, his alcohol intake is less or "a few" beers a day.

1. What additional pain assessment information should be obtained?

2. How would you propose this patient's pain should be managed at this time?

3. If this patient's physician is reluctant to prescribe opioid analgesics to adequately manage the pain, what resources or help might you turn to?

4. What non-pharmacologic approaches are appropriate to implement in this situation?

Case Study #5 Answers

1.   **Answer**: Careful assessment of his pain is needed. Elicit a description of the pain—aching, burning, sharp, dull, etc. When is it worse; when is it better? Is one position better than another? What is the current prescribed pain regimen? Does he drink to alleviate the pain? What over-the-counter medications has he tried to help with pain? Has he ever been on methadone or any other prescription medication for pain or addiction? Has he ever been in a rehab program?

2.   **Answer**: The best recommendation is to start by assuring the patient that you are committed to helping him get pain relief. What is an acceptable level of relief? Let the patient know that you will help him obtain relief so that he doesn't have to drink to relieve pain. Discuss the dangers of mixing strong pain medications and alcohol. Increase his current opioid regimen if necessary and add an adjuvant analgesic for bone pain (e.g., ibuprofen 400-600 mg TID) and ask him and his caregivers to keep a log of medication administration as well as self-pain rating. Ensure that medications are given as scheduled with breakthrough medication as needed. Ensure that you start a program for prevention of constipation. Know that a patient with a history of substance abuse may require higher than usual doses of medication to receive relief.

3.   **Answer**: Radiation therapy, if he hasn't had any; higher doses of adjuvant medications (NSAIDs, steroids); intervention by the social worker to evaluate if there are issues the patient has used alcohol to hide.

4.   **Answer**:
     a.   Music therapy consult, chaplain support, directed visualization/relaxation
     b.   Distraction, i.e., funny videos, action movies, etc.

Case Study #6a

You are the case manager for an 85-year-old woman, Agnes, who has breast cancer metastatic to the bone, brain and liver. Her present pain regimen is long-acting, oral morphine 120 mg/day with 5 mg short-acting morphine for breakthrough pain. Her primary caregiver is her 87-year-old frail husband, Will. They have lived in a retirement apartment community for several years and have many friends who are already grieving the loss of their dear friend. Agnes and Will are devoted to one another, having been married for nearly 65 years and never have been apart for more than a day. Their three children live out of state but come every month or so to visit and help. Lately, Will is having an increasingly difficult time keeping medications straight and Agnes is often in pain, unable to sleep at night. Several friends who are retired nurses have tried to help, but have warned Will about the "dangerous" medications Agnes is taking. He has called you because he wants Agnes off all of her pain medications, saying, "She was much better before she started with hospice." When you arrive at their home, you observe Will unshaven and overly tired. The apartment is cluttered with laundry, dirty dishes and old newspapers. Both Will and Agnes tearfully tell you they cannot go on much longer. Agnes rates her pain as a "10" on a 0-10 scale.

1. There are many issues/needs in this situation. List them. What is your first priority? Why?

2. Is there additional assessment information you need?

3. How should you, as the hospice nurse, approach them in an effort to achieve better control of Agnes' pain?

4. What might you recommend for Agnes' pain management regimen?

Case Study #6a Answers

1. **Answer**: Uncontrolled pain, poor understanding of pain control, exhausted caregiver, "well-meaning" friends who are uneducated about pain management, poor understanding of disease progression, patient/husband fear of separation from each other, "inadequate" caregiver. First priority is pain control. Patient and husband will both benefit if the pain is controlled. Other issues can be dealt with when pain is controlled.

2. **Answer**: A thorough pain assessment, including descriptions of the pain, duration, aggravating/relieving factors, etc., should be elicited. How often is the short-acting morphine being used? What other medications is the patient taking, if any, for pain or other symptoms or side effects? Also, a thorough assessment of caregiving resources should be conducted.

3. **Answer**: The approach needs to be gentle and both must feel supported. The husband needs to understand that some of his wife's symptoms are due to progression of her illness and that he can best show his love for her by helping her to be comfortable. If she is comfortable, she may be able to sleep better and so will he. She may also be better able to participate in her ADLs, further decreasing the burden on him. He needs to learn the importance of caring for himself, so he can be there for his wife; and to know that those who care about he and his wife can help him with the burden of caregiving. A home health aide should be recommended. Continuous care, if available, would be helpful for pain management and teaching. Respite care could also be offered to provide the husband with a break from caregiving and for needed rest.

4. **Answer**: Once the patient's pain has been adequately controlled on oral morphine, this is a situation where transdermal fentanyl would be a good choice as a long-acting medication since she is not opioid-naïve and her oral doses are becoming higher. Fentanyl would decrease the husband's burden/responsibility in administering more frequent oral medications while giving the patient an excellent base of pain relief. Friends may be less concerned about a patch than high oral doses of medication. The appropriate starting dose would be a 50 mcg/hr patch (½ daily dose of oral morphine would be 60 mg and patches are available in 50 and 75 mg). The existing breakthrough dose is inadequate and needs to be adjusted (10-15% of 120 mg/day would be 12-18 mg every 2 hours so the short-acting morphine should probably be dosed at 15 mg rather than 5 mg). Adjuvant medications, particularly an NSAID for bone pain and/or an antidepressant/anticonvulsant if neuropathic pain is present should also be considered.

Case Study #6b

You are the case manager for an 85-year-old woman, Agnes, who has breast cancer metastatic to the bone, brain and liver. Her present pain regimen is long-acting, oral morphine 120 mg/day with 5 mg short-acting morphine for breakthrough pain. Her primary caregiver is her 87-year-old frail husband, Will. They have lived in a retirement apartment community for several years and have many friends who are already grieving the loss of their dear friend. Agnes and Will are devoted to one another, having been married for nearly 65 years and never have been apart for more than a day. Their three children live out of state but come every month or so to visit and help. Lately, Will is having an increasingly difficult time keeping medications straight and Agnes is often in pain, unable to sleep at night. Several friends who are retired nurses have tried to help, but have warned Will about the "dangerous" medications Agnes is taking. He has called you because he wants Agnes off all of her pain medications, saying, "She was much better before she started with hospice." When you arrive at their home, you observe Will unshaven and overly tired. The apartment is cluttered with laundry, dirty dishes and old newspapers. Both Will and Agnes tearfully tell you they cannot go on much longer. Agnes rates her pain as a "10" on a 0-10 scale.

5.   What non-pharmacologic approaches are appropriate to implement in this situation?

6.   How can the other members of the interdisciplinary team be helpful with Agnes and Will?

7.   Consider how hospices define "family." Who are Agnes and Will's "family"? How can (or should) the hospice team support and educate them?

Case Study #6b Answers

5. **Answer**: Hospice social worker as well as all staff can help the husband to understand his losses and fears related to her disease and impending death and how important it is that they have quality time together until her death.

6. **Answer**: Volunteer manager and chaplain can be involved to direct friends and family as well as provide respite care. Home health aide can be assigned. Respite or continuous care nurses can be instituted for a short time until pain is under control.

7. **Answer**: Hospice IDTs usually define "family" as those who are important to the patient. In this case, their friends in the retirement community are as much "family" as any blood relatives. If Will and Agnes wish these friends to help with care, it would be appropriate for them to have some training from the hospice nurse and/or volunteer coordinator.

Case Study #7a

You have arrived at JG's house. He has a hospice diagnosis of small cell lung cancer with diffuse metastasis to the bone. He complains of severe shortness of breath, but does not have a cardiac history. His caregiver tells you that lately he has had a tendency to get a little anxious at times. And lately he has become intermittently forgetful and confused. When you arrive you note his vital signs to be BP: 158/88 AR: 124 RR: 26 T: 99°F.

His current medications include

      Sustained-release morphine 60 mg PO every 12 hours
      Immediate release morphine 15 mg PO every 3 hours PRN
      Paroxetine HCl 10 mg PO every day
      Albuterol sulfate/ipratropium bromide 1 vial via nebulizer every 4 hours while awake
      Salmeterol inhaler 2 puffs BID
      Lorazepam 0.5 mg 1 PO every 6 hours PRN
      Guaifenesin sustained release 600 mg PO BID

1.   What key pieces of information will you include in your assessment?

Case Study #7a Answers

1. **Answer: Assessment can include**

   - Anxiety level?
   - Does the lorazepam help?
   - How often does he take lorazepam?
   - Are inhalers used effectively (have the patient demonstrate self administration)?
   - Do the inhalers help shortness of breath?
   - Does the patient have oxygen?
   - What is the liter flow?
   - Does the patient have increased respiratory secretions?
   - Does the immediate release morphine help with shortness of breath?
   - How much immediate release morphine is JG using in 24 hours?
   - Does JG use his medications as prescribed? If not, why not?
   - Do you have a documented pain assessment? Is pain related to anxiety? Shortness of breath?
   - When is the onset and what is the duration of shortness of breath?
   - What is the lung assessment?
   - Have you done a bowel assessment?
   - Is the patient impacted?
   - Why is there no bowel regimen ordered?
   - Mental status?

Case Study #7b

You have arrived at JG's house. He has a hospice diagnosis of small cell lung cancer with diffuse metastasis to the bone. He complains of severe shortness of breath, but does not have a cardiac history. His caregiver tells you that lately he has had a tendency to get a little anxious at times. And lately he has become intermittently forgetful and confused. When you arrive you note his vital signs to be BP: 158/88 AR: 124 RR: 26 T: 99°F.

His current medications include
Sustained-release morphine 60 mg PO every 12 hours
Immediate release morphine 15 mg PO every 3 hours PRN
Paroxetine HCl 10 mg PO every day
Albuterol sulfate/ipratropium bromide 1 vial via nebulizer every 4 hours while awake
Salmeterol inhaler 2 puffs BID
Lorazepam 0.5 mg 1 PO every 6 hours PRN
Guaifenesin sustained release 600 mg PO BID

2.   What should be the nurse's first response?

Case Study #7b Answers

2.   **Answer:** The shortness of breath needs to be dealt with immediately. Assist the patient into a high-Fowler's position, encourage pursed lip breathing and aim a fan at the patient's face. Consider a trial of oxygen; following lung assessment is it possible the patient has an accumulation of fluid? Pneumonia? Would thoracentesis or antibiotics be indicated? Anxiety and pain can play a role in shortness of breath issues. Look at breaking the cycle of anxiety/pain/dyspnea in the team approach to care. Ensure that all are well controlled. Management of bone pain should include an NSAID, which is missing from JG's pain regimen.

The increase in confusion needs to be explored. Possible etiologies include polypharmacy, hypoxemia, brain metastases, and hypercalcemia. Are there any medications that could be eliminated from the regimen? Lorazepam? Can another anti-anxiety agent be as effective without amnesic effects? The patient may benefit from radiation therapy or steroids for the management of the brain metastases.

With respect to hypercalcemia, a calcium level should be drawn if the patient is at a point in the disease when treatment would still be considered. A high level of serum calcium is considered to be greater than 11mEq/L. Serum calcium levels alone do not always give a true picture. Calcium levels must be adjusted using serum albumin levels to determine a corrected serum calcium level. A low albumin level common in patients with advanced disease gives a false low calcium level. A serum level of 16 mEq/L is an ominous number and without aggressive treatment the symptoms are often irreversible. Symptoms that are common are: drowsiness, stupor, coma, nausea, vomiting, polyuria, thirst, dehydration, constipation, fatigue, muscular weakness, diminished deep tendon reflexes, anorexia, paralytic ileus, and seizures. If hypercalcemia were present it would be important to clarify goals of treatment with JG and his family. Treat the underlying cause if appropriate and treat the symptoms. Early treatments include hydration and diuresis. Pamidronate sodium 60-90 mg given IV in one infusion is recommended treatment for moderate to severe hypercalcemia and relatively easy to administer.

Case Study #7c

You have arrived at JG's house. He has a hospice diagnosis of small cell lung cancer with diffuse metastasis to the bone. He complains of severe shortness of breath, but does not have a cardiac history. His caregiver tells you that lately he has had a tendency to get a little anxious at times. And lately he has become intermittently forgetful and confused. When you arrive you note his vital signs to be BP: 158/88 AR: 124 RR: 26 T: 99°F.

His current medications include
> Sustained-release morphine 60 mg PO every 12 hours
> Immediate release morphine 15 mg PO every 3 hours PRN
> Paroxetine HCl 10 mg PO every day
> Albuterol sulfate/ipratropium bromide 1 vial via nebulizer every 4 hours while awake
> Salmeterol inhaler 2 puffs BID
> Lorazepam 0.5 mg 1 PO every 6 hours PRN
> Guaifenesin sustained release 600 mg PO BID

3.   What other needs should be addressed?

Case Study #7c Answers

3. **Answer:** Constipation and impaction can be a factor in a patient's increasing confusion and is also a symptom of hypercalcemia. A bowel assessment and regimen are critical for this patient.

The other important component of care for this person is the role of the various members of the inter-disciplinary team (IDT). Psychosocial, spiritual, functional, and physical needs of the patient and family should all be addressed and included in the plan of care. One should also look at the complementary therapies and how they may improve the care of this patient. Massage therapy for relaxation and energy work, music therapy for relaxation and refocusing, aromatherapy for relaxation and stress relief, also homeopathic remedies, and supplements are often used. When the complements are added to conventional medical care, the results can be impressive. They must be used appropriately with attention to cultural considerations and ensuring that the physician/pharmacist is aware of any substances being used which could interact with prescribed medications.

Case Study #8a

KC is a 36-year-old woman with a diagnosis of colon cancer with multiple sites of metastatic disease to the liver and lymph nodes. When you arrive at her home her husband and 2 children are present. You learn that she has been lethargic and confused at times. She has had surgery and chemotherapy (last treatment 3 months ago). On your assessment you identify

- Recent mild nausea
- Poor appetite
- No BM for 4 days
- C/o lower back pain visual analog scale = 6/10 not relieved by oxycodone 5 mg/acetaminophen 500 mg of which she takes 2 caps every 3 hours around the clock
- Functional status Karnofsky score of 50
- The rectal vault is empty and she has rare, sluggish bowel sounds
- You note evidence of ascites, hepatomegaly and a tender lower abdomen
- She is jaundiced and her skin is cool and clammy
- She appears frightened, confused and clumsy. She is not able to perform the elements of the Mini Mental Status Exam
- BP 110/54 HR 104 RR 24 T 99

Her current medications include
    Psyllium
    Metoclopramide hydrochloride
    Lorazepam
    Fluoxetine hydrochloride
    Megestrol acetate
    Oxycodone 5 mg/ acetaminophen 500 mg

1. What is the main issue in this situation?

2. What interventions/actions would you take in regards to her confusion and lethargy? What recommendations would you make? What should be the nurse's first response?

3. What interventions/actions would you take in regards to her pain? What recommendations would you make? What should be the nurse's first response?

Case Study #8a Answers

1. **Answer:** There are many issues present in this case. First, consider disease progression in metastatic colon cancer. The issues of pain, intestinal obstruction, ascites and high ammonia levels are common in advanced disease states where hepatic metastases are present. The patient's disease is obviously advancing. Which of her symptoms can be better managed through assessment and interventions? Certainly her constipation and potential for obstruction should be assessed along with her increased lethargy and confusion.

2. **Answer**: High ammonia levels are common in liver disease; more often associated with cirrhosis of the liver, but can be seen in metastatic disease to the liver such as in KC's case. Lactulose is the drug of choice as it is metabolized by gut bacteria to acetic and lactic acids, which prevent bacterial conversion of urea to ammonia. Lactulose causes diarrhea, thus reducing ammonia levels. Cardinal signs of increase ammonia levels are confusion, profound lethargy, alterations in consciousness levels; jaundice is usually present, tremors, as well as cool and clammy skin. High ammonia levels can be a terminal event, without treatment. Sleep and obtundation come quickly. Treatment may be appropriate in this case and lactulose may have some benefit in treating constipation as well.

3. **Answer**: KC has rated her pain at 6 on the numeric intensity scale. Her total daily intake equals 80 mg of oxycodone + 8000 mg of acetaminophen. This dose is 4000 mg over the recommended ceiling dose of acetaminophen. In the presence of liver disease this is a critical dose and could be contributing to her liver failure. Therefore, her oxycodone/acetaminophen should be changed to oxycodone alone with the possible addition of an NSAID. Her current daily dose of oxycodone should be given in 4 hour increments (80/6 = 14) so an appropriate starting dose would be 15-20 mg every 4 hours since she is not in pain control. If we start at 15 mg every 4 hours, then her total daily dose of oxycodone would be 90 mg. An appropriate breakthrough dose (10-15% of 24-hour dose given orally every 2 hours) would be 10-15 mg of oxycodone every two hours. Good pain management is about assessment and re-assessment. The use of non-pharmacologic interventions should be considered and encouraged. After symptom management is addressed, advance directives and DNR status need to be discussed since the patient's disease has progressed.

Case Study #8b

KC is a 36-year-old woman with a diagnosis of colon cancer with multiple sites of metastatic disease to the liver and lymph nodes. When you arrive at her home her husband and two children are present. You learn that she has been lethargic and confused at times. She has had surgery and chemotherapy (last treatment three months ago). On your assessment you identify

- Recent mild nausea
- Poor appetite
- No BM for 4 days
- C/o lower back pain visual analog scale = 6/10 not relieved by oxycodone 5 mg/acetaminophen 500 mg of which she takes 2 caps every 3 hours around the clock
- Functional status Karnofsky score of 50
- The rectal vault is empty and she has rare, sluggish bowel sounds
- You note evidence of ascites, hepatomegaly and a tender lower abdomen
- She is jaundiced and her skin is cool and clammy
- She appears frightened, confused and clumsy. She is not able to perform the elements of the Mini Mental Status Exam
- BP 110/54 HR 104 RR 24 T 99

Her current medications include
    Psyllium
    Metoclopramide hydrochloride
    Lorazepam
    Fluoxetine hydrochloride
    Megestrol acetate
    Oxycodone 5 mg/ acetaminophen 500 mg

4.   What interventions/actions would you take in regards to her bowels and other GI symptoms? What recommendations would you make? What should be the nurse's first response?

5.   What other needs should be addressed?

Cast Study #8b Answers

4. **Answer:** Assessment reveals no BM for 4 days, poor appetite and nausea. Her skin is cool and clammy. She is hypotensive with an increased heart rate; rectal vault is empty and ballooned, with rare sluggish bowel sounds. Ascites and distention are present; she has low back pain and abdominal tenderness on palpation. She has not eaten in days. This may be a picture of bowel obstruction. Bowel obstruction occurs most commonly in ovarian and colon cancers. Occasionally it may occur in malignancies such as endometrial, prostate, lymphomas, bladder, and stomach. Symptoms can include continuous pain, nausea, vomiting, constipation, diarrhea, colicky pain, anorexia, and confusion. An empty ballooned rectum on rectal exam can be a sign of impaction with feces higher up in the colon. Since severe constipation can mimic obstruction, the exam is important. The treatment for constipation is a stool softener and a stimulant. Bisacodyl tablets and an enema are appropriate here, with a timely reassessment of results. Psyllium is a poor choice for KC as it may add bulk to her stool and prevent evacuation from a lack of fluids intake. Her bowel regimen has been weak, as she has been taking opioids for pain. The rule of thumb is that patients on opioids should begin a bowel regimen with a softener and a bowel stimulant. Lactulose will also be added to her regimen. Metoclopramide should be discontinued if obstruction is possible since it increases motility in the upper GI tract.

    It is important to know the etiology of nausea. Is the vomiting center being affected via the CTZ? Vestibular apparatus? Cerebral cortex? or Vagal stimulus? Each type of nausea requires a different approach. Prochlorperazine, dexamethasone and metoclopramide (in the ABSENCE of obstruction) are all appropriate choices. The megestrol acetate should also be discontinued after discussion with the family. With disease progression, GI symptoms and lethargy/confusion, megestrol acetate is not appropriate at this time to increase weight gain and appetite stimulation.

5. **Answer:** Education and preparation of the family for the patient's declining functional status and death should be addressed. Teaching regarding disease progression, symptoms, and symptom management and indicators of imminent death are all warranted at this time. Assessing the family's awareness and preparation as well as addressing advance directives are all appropriate interventions. Psychosocial and spiritual interventions should be offered as well.

Case Study #9

     Mr. L is a 54-year-old man with amyotrophic lateral sclerosis (ALS). He was diagnosed 6 years ago and has been receiving care at home. He is bedridden at home on BiPAP and receives frequent suctioning. He has devoted caregivers and his skin is intact without any bedsores. When he begins to have more periods of distress, his caregivers suggest a palliative care team consult. Medications include lorazepam for anxiety and sensations of breathlessness.

1.   What medications would you suggest for emergency episodes of dyspnea? What route? What dose?

2.   When the patient has more difficulty breathing, what would recommendations be?

3.   If the patient would like to get longer acting benzodiazepine, what would you suggest?

4.   Since the patient is bed bound, what other issues would be important?

5.   What would be important issues to educate his family around his death?

6.   What could you do for thickened saliva?

7.   What medications would be helpful if you want to dry up secretions?

Case Study #9 Answers

1. **Answer**: Morphine elixir PO/sublingual 5-15 mg every 1 hour or 1-4 mg subcutaneous every 30 minutes as needed

2. **Answer**: Titrate opioids upwards as needed to control breathlessness while carefully monitoring patient.

3. **Answer**: Diazepam 5-10 mg every 6-8 hours

4. **Answer**: Bowel regimen, skin care and sleep schedule due to inactivity

5. **Answer**: Anticipatory education for a respiratory death including fear, anxiety, escalating respiratory distress—all symptoms will be managed. Advanced Care Planning around comfort care should be discussed including discussion of the benefits/burdens of intubation, feeding tubes, antibiotics, and management of other common symptoms and relevant concerns in ALS at advanced stages.

6. **Answer**: Guaifenesin long acting 600 mg every 12 hours

7. **Answer**: Any of the following medications would be helpful
   - Scopolamine
   - Hyoscyamine
   - Atropine
   - DiphenhydrAMINE

Case Study #10

Ms. A is a 43-year-old with end stage HIV/AIDS. She has had HIV for 6-7 years. Illnesses have included bouts of pneumocystis carinii pneumonia (PCP), cryptococcal meningitis, cervical cancer, myobacterium avilum intracellular (MAI) complex. More recently, she has had seizures and has been referred for palliative care following a diagnosis of progressive multifocal leukoencephalopathy (PML). Currently, her CD4 count is 16. She is no longer taking antiretrovirals, however remains on antibiotics for C. diff and fungemia. She also has a history of drug abuse and pain management has been an issue.

1. What are some issues to be addressed in terms of long-term care?

2. In assessing pain, what would be important elements to consider?

3. How would pain be addressed in response to her history of addiction?

4. What is difference between addiction and tolerance?

Case Study #10 Answers

1. **Answer**: Advanced Care Planning including DNR/DNI. Where does she want to die? What is her support system? Is there a primary caregiver? What are the possible settings of care for her as the disease advances?

2. **Answer**: The typical assessment, which would include, location, duration, intensity, factors which increase or decrease pain, other medications currently prescribed. A description of the pain would be particularly helpful in differentiating pain types and appropriate medication regimens, especially since neuropathic pain is common in patients with HIV disease.

3. **Answer**: Separate pain from any methadone maintenance program. May need to contract with the program for medications.

4. **Answer**: Addiction is a primary, chronic, neurobiologic disease, with genetic, psychosocial and environmental factors influencing its development and manifestations. It is characterized by behaviors that include one or more of the following: impaired control over drug use, compulsive use continued despite harm and craving. Tolerance is a state of adaptation in which exposure to a drug induces changes that result in a diminution of one or more of the drug's effects over time.

Case Study #11

Ms. N is a 43-year-old woman with end stage renal failure and peripheral vascular disease. She was admitted for surgery of a non-healing ulcer of her left foot. Post-operatively she developed an infection necessitating a left below knee amputation (BKA). Then complications arose with her right leg and she underwent a right BKA. Soon thereafter, she developed gangrene. Ms. N is now considering whether to undergo more surgery or discontinue all aggressive measures including her dialysis.

1. What pain control should be initiated for painful dressing changes?

2. What dosing adjustments must be considered with her renal failure?

3. If she forgoes dialysis, what would her course be?

4. What adjustments would be necessary for her pain control?

5. What family education regarding her death is necessary?

Case Study #11 Answers

1. **Answer:** The patient should receive intravenous pain medication (morphine or hydromorphone) 15-30 minutes prior to dressing changes.

2. **Answer:** Dosing should take into account altered metabolism and excretion due to renal failure, so doses may be lower than usual to start, with slower titration and longer intervals. Assess pain and sedation levels frequently to determine effectiveness and under/overdosing.

3. **Answer:** Usually death occurs within 7-10 days. Patients may be responsive the first 3-4 days and then slowly progress into a coma. It depends somewhat on Ms. N's current BUN, creatinine, and potassium levels but with advanced renal failure coupled with gangrene, her decline will no doubt be rapid and progressive. Uremia will occur which may result in severe pruritus. Metabolic acidosis will result in confusion, stupor, possible seizures, and coma.

4. **Answer:** Ms. N. will need good pain control due to the gangrene and adjuvants may be indicated to manage itching, and confusion. Anticonvulsants should be readily available since seizures are a possibility. However, much less medication is needed since it will not leave the body once dialysis is stopped. Careful dosing is important due to her altered metabolism.

5. **Answer:** Describe the renal death as above. The family needs an estimated time frame so that they can prepare emotionally, spiritually, and financially. They need to be assured that symptoms such as pain, itching, fever, agitation/confusion, and/or seizures will be adequately managed and that the patient will slip into a coma and the death will likely be peaceful. Funeral planning support should be offered through members of the interdisciplinary team.

Case Study #12

Mr. L is a 55-year-old male with end-stage cardiomyopathy. His ejection fraction is 10%. He has undergone all possible surgical interventions without improvement. He is currently on a dobutamine drip that is maintaining his blood pressure. He would like to go home to die.

1.   What would the discharge plan be?

2.   What would you give for chest pain?

3.   What other medications would be important?

4.   What patient/family education is important?

Case Study #12 Answers

1. **Answer**: The patient and family should be given the option of continuing the dobutamine at least long enough to get him home and settled in. He will need someone with him at all times, so that his exertion is minimal. Oxygen, diuretics, antianxiety, and pain medicines are all indicated. Once at home the dobutamine can be discontinued and opioids initiated.

2. **Answer**: Morphine, as it will also ease dyspnea and air hunger.

3. **Answer**: Primarily benzodiazepines as in the emergency room a patient is treated with opioids and benzodiazepines so this should be simulated at home. Diuretics, digoxin (if patient opts to continue it), antianxiety medications such as lorazepam and perhaps a sleeping medication.

4. **Answer**: Family needs to know possible scenarios with this patient, especially the most likely one of pulmonary edema/respiratory distress and/or pneumonia. Discussion should take place about which medications will be used. For some families, oral antibiotics are seen as comfort medications. Otherwise, they need assurance that medicines such as morphine or hydromorphone and diazepam or lorazepam should be given every 15 minutes until comfort is attained. The goal is to assure the patient will not experience any distress and that death will be peaceful and gradual or could come as the result of a sudden event (PE, MI, etc.).

Case Study #13

Ms. S is a 21-year-old young woman status post multiple liver transplants. Her liver failure began when she was 13. She has undergone two liver transplants. The first one failed three years after the transplant. She is on numerous immunosuppressive medications and states her quality of life is poor and she doesn't want to live like this anymore. She has decided to stop all of her medications.

1.   What assessment is necessary of Ms. S and her family?

2.   What medications are appropriate for treatment of Ms. S?

3.   What information should be given to the family about what Ms. S may experience in her dying process? What preparation hints would you give?

Case Study #13 Answers

1. **Answer:** It is necessary to assess for depression and if indicated decision-making capacity. Treatment for depression should be instituted. If it is determined she lacks capacity to make decisions, then it would be important to determine her identified decision maker for healthcare issues, or closest family member and any other advance directives. This decision maker would then be responsible for making her healthcare decisions, including choices about continuing her immunosuppressive regimen or not. If she clearly has capacity and she is not depressed, then her choices to discontinue medications should be honored.

2. **Answer:** Ms. S will need medication for pain such as morphine, hydromorphone or oxycodone, for urticaria such as antihistamines, hydrocortisone lotion or other medications, for fever such as indomethacin suppositories or other liquid NSAIDS, for dyspnea such as opioids, for agitation and for hallucinations from encephalopathy such as haloperidol or chlorpromazine.

3. **Answer:** The family should be told, gently, that death could follow a lapse into a coma and be peaceful or could occur suddenly as the result of internal bleeding. They should also be told that confusion/agitation and pain are possibilities when dealing with hepatic failure. The family should be guided to have dark towels available in the event of a massive GI bleed. They should be given instructions on how to administer prefilled syringes of morphine and diazepam in the event of a sudden bleed to assure comfort and explain these will not prolong or hasten her life but make sure she has no distress.

Case Study #14

E.L. is an 11-year-old Cambodian boy living in the northern United States who experienced an anoxic brain injury at the age of 6. He was involved in an accident where he fell under ice for 45 minutes resulting in respiratory arrest. He was found unresponsive. He continued to be unresponsive following pulmonary resuscitation and has lived in a rehabilitation setting in a permanent vegetative state. He has been developing recurrent pneumonias necessitating hospitalizations and aggressive respiratory therapy. Recently, the family has decided his quality of life is poor and they want no further antibiotic therapy.

1. What assessment of the patient and family is indicated?

2. What assessment of the staff is necessary?

3. What signs and symptoms would be attended to in making this boy more comfortable?

4. What medications are necessary to treat these symptoms?

5. What family/staff education is important in this scenario?

Case Study #14 Answers

1. **Answer:** One needs to assess whether there is a language barrier and find an interpreter if necessary to convene a family meeting. During this time, one needs to first explore the cultural implications of the death of a young boy and any religious beliefs that are important to this process. Then one needs to ensure that the family understands the outcome of foregoing antibiotics. They should also be assured any subsequent symptoms that occur will be aggressively managed. Finally, if appropriate, the family may want to understand the dying process. The team should explore the spiritual/religious support needed in this case.

2. **Answer:** The staff has become extended family. They need to be given ample opportunity to process the parent's decision and the parent's right to choose this option. It would be good to give detailed explanations of the scenarios that are possible for the boy and how symptoms will be managed. It is important for the palliative care team to allow those uncomfortable with this to support their conscientious objection. Finally, it needs to be impressed upon staff that care has not been withdrawn; rather there is more intensive detail to symptoms. Perhaps, to get buy-in, it would be best to use medications that are currently being used and not withdraw all treatments at once.

3. **Answer:** This child will likely experience fever, sweats, dyspnea, and increased upper airway secretions.

4. **Answer:** Treat the fever with acetaminophen or indomethacin suppositories, as they are longer acting. Treat dyspnea with opioids or nebulized medications such as albuterol or steroids if that is what he has been consistently receiving. For congestion, glycopyrrolate nebulizer treatments, scopolamine, or even IV diphenhydrAMINE can help. Finally, IV fluids should be discontinued or decreased to a keep vein open level.

5. **Answer:** Family needs to be assured of non-abandonment, adequate symptom management and preservation of dignity. They need to be offered information and allowed to make choices. Again cultural and spiritual assessment is critical to assure respect and support. Staff needs to be supported through the process. Frequent staff assessment and debriefing after the death may be necessary. It is also important to consider any siblings in the plan of care.

Case Study #15a

A 33-year-old Muslim woman from Republic of Mali is diagnosed with widespread, advanced ovarian cancer. She has received surgery and chemotherapy but her disease has progressed. She and her husband have been in America for 5 years having come to work and send money home to Africa to support family. She does not speak English and through the use of telephone language line interpreters, staff is informed that she wishes to delegate all decisions to her husband. The interpreter is asked to explore the patient's understanding of her illness and reports that in her culture it is not appropriate to ask or to tell a person that they are seriously ill and might die of their disease. Both patient and husband expect expert input and treatment from the doctor rather than being engaged in collaborative decision-making. Her husband is incredulous that in America this disease cannot be treated further or cured. The husband cannot talk openly about the potential that his wife may die as acknowledging this is considered a challenge to the will of Allah. No one knows who will live and who will die.

1. How might the palliative care or hospice team begin its assessment and development of an appropriate plan of care for this family?

2. What are the issues that will require particular awareness and sensitivity from the staff?

3. How can the team help each other to meet the needs of this family?

Case Study #15a Answers

1. **Answer:** The preliminary assessment has yielded important information about decision-making and expectations of the healthcare team. This information should be comprehended by the team before taking the assessment further. A comprehensive assessment should be completed, with particular attention to the family's expectations from the hospice/palliative care team, needs and preferences for care at home if that is the setting of choice and how communication will be handled to ensure that the language barrier is minimized. Assessment questions may be addressed to the patient to gather data, but items needing decision should be addressed to the husband per the patient's request. The team should recognize that the husband, while unable to talk about the expected death of the patient, should be given the opportunity to vent and grieve his losses of the health of his wife and his frustration with the lack of treatment. Psychosocial needs and spiritual needs of the patient and family should not be neglected despite the cultural differences.

2. **Answer:** The team should know and recognize the areas of healthcare where they may find differences resulting from cultural and/or religious beliefs and values that should be noted and incorporated into the plan of care. These are special areas of attention: time orientation; emphasis on past versus present or future; decision making style; self-determination/autonomy versus family, community decision making; ideas about the causation of illness; preferences and comfort with concept of "advance care planning"; appropriateness of clothing, food preferences; traditional remedies; issues related to privacy, gender, eye contact, personal space; communication styles and preferences: truth telling, direct, non-verbal, respect for silence; taboos, rituals and healing practices; treatment decisions such as nutrition/hydration, discontinuing treatments, organ donation; customs and beliefs related to death, transitions, after-life; expectations and perceptions of healthcare relationships i.e., egalitarian, hierarchical, informal, or paternalistic; practices and behaviors related to illness, pain, treatments, suffering and end of life.

    By asking general, open ended questions about the family's cultural practices/beliefs, the team will gather information helpful to them in meeting the patient and family needs, while avoiding a direct discussion of death and funeral preparations.

3. **Answer:** The patient and family will be best served by a team with good communication and trust where the members are able to challenge each other when making unintended assumptions or demonstrating bias without awareness.

Case Study #15b

As the patient's death nears, the staff continues to request the husband's input in providing care which meets the family's needs and preferences. Staff insures that the patient is facing east toward Mecca and understands the importance of the prayers and verses from the Qur'an that are valued ritual at the time of death. There can be no planning for a funeral until, after the death and at that time, only family or Muslim staff can care for the body. Her husband and friends from the mosque will wash and dress the body in an unsewn white cloth.

4. What additional information does the staff need to know in order to provide care and support to the family at the time of death?

5. What teaching needs to be done with the husband, family and friends?

Case Study #15b Answers

4. **Answer:** The team needs to know whether the nurse will be able to touch the patient to pronounce the patient dead. The team will need to communicate what the basic laws are that need to be respected while ensuring respect for their cultural beliefs. The team should explain what would be required if death does occur in terms of pronouncement, notification of the physician, completion of the death certificate, disposal of controlled substances, etc., while respecting the cultural preferences regarding preparation of the body. The team also needs to know plans regarding use of a funeral home or not and if any special preferences need to be communicated in advance to the mortuary.

5. **Answer:** In addition to the explanations listed above, the team should not neglect to prepare the family and friends in attendance what is expected as death draws near. If the team cannot refer to the patient's expected death, they could talk about what would happen if a patient in this condition were to die, or discuss what has happened in similar cases so as not to violate religious practices. The team needs to ensure that the family knows not to call for emergency services and transport but to contact the palliative care/hospice team as this will ensure that their preferences and individualized care plan will be carried out. The team must also do teaching with any staff who may serve this patient/family at the time of death to ensure that preferences are understood.

Case Study #16

Bill is a 71-year-old patient who is dying in the hospital of metastatic lung cancer. He has been in severe neuropathic pain during his illness and has received multiple interventions including anesthetic procedures (blocks) and intraspinal medications. His tumor has affected the brachial plexus and his pain continues to increase as he nears death despite the best efforts of the pain resource team, oncology team and palliative care team. His family has requested sedation for the intractable pain. They can no longer bear to see him suffer.

1.   What actions does the team need to take to ensure the appropriateness of this intervention?

Case Study #16 Answer

1. **Answer:** The team needs to make sure that all reasonable efforts to address the patient's pain have been taken, including all appropriate consultations, and second opinions. The team should examine the patient's history, disease progression, and other available diagnostic information to ensure that no treatable etiology or cause that can be otherwise managed has been missed. The patient should be involved in the discussion of actions and interventions if he has capacity. If not, the patient's healthcare proxy or decision-maker should be fully informed that the goal of the sedation is for patient comfort and not to hasten death, although this is a potential unintended outcome. The medical record should clearly document the review of the patient's history and interventions, the team discussion, the discussions with patient and family, and the actions taken.

Pharmacology

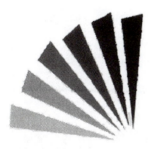

Medication Questions

1. Combination analgesics that contain acetaminophen are not recommended for patients with hepatic insufficiency. What is the recommended alternative?

2. What is the maximum recommended number of milligrams of acetaminophen permitted per day?

3. If 20 mg of oxycodone is equivalent to 30 mg morphine then how much morphine is equivalent to 60 mg of oxycodone?

4. You are called to consult on a new patient who will be discharged home. You are asked to convert her morphine infusion to oral medications. Presently, her pain is well controlled with morphine 7 mg/hour by SQ infusion.

    A. What dose of long-acting morphine would you recommend?

    B. What is the appropriate medication for breakthrough pain? What dose would you recommend?

    C. What would you recommend for the dose of fentanyl? What medications are most appropriate for breakthrough pain with transdermal fentanyl?

    D. What else should be considered when starting a patient on a transdermal patch?

1. Answer: Acetaminophen or an NSAID should be dosed separately from the opioid analgesic, which should be given as a single agent. This allows individual titration of each drug to effect without side effects related to one drug. Acetaminophen should be used cautiously in persons with altered liver function.

2. Answer: 4000 mg or 4 G Acetaminophen should also be used cautiously in persons with impaired liver function.

3. Answer: 60 (current dose)/20 (current equivalent) x 30 (new equivalent) = 90 mg

4. Answers

   A. 7 mg x 24 hours = 168 mg morphine IV/SQ 168 mg/10 x 30 = 504 mg oral dose equivalent for 24 hours or 250 mg PO every 12 hours. Could be dosed at 230 mg or 260 mg for ease of administration with available dosages (100 mg x 2 plus 30 mg or 60 mg)

   B. Morphine is the correct medication for breakthrough pain. The recommended dose for breakthrough would be 10-15% (or up to 20%) of 500 mg or 50-75 mg (100 mg) every 1-2 hours PO PRN. This could be easily dosed with tablets at 60 mg.

   C. Transdermal fentanyl is 50% of the daily dose of morphine or 250 mcg/hr. Breakthrough dose is approximately Z\c of the mcg/hr dose, 80 mg of morphine PO every 1-2 hours PRN. In tablets, this would be most appropriately dosed at 60 mg since pain is well-controlled but could go up to 90 mg if needed. Oxycodone 40 mg or hydromorphone 15 mg could also be used.

   D. The patient and family need to be instructed that it takes 48-72 hours for the patch to reach effectiveness and that short-term analgesia (morphine) needs to be taken every four hours until the transdermal fentanyl is effective (500 mg total 24-hour dose/6 doses = approx. 80 mg every 4 hours PO which could be dosed at 60 or 90 mg). Hospice staff should closely monitor patient's pain control and medication side effects in the first critical days after the medication changeover.

5.   The only NSAID available for parenteral administration is

   A.   Naproxen

   B.   Sulindac

   C.   Ibuprofen

   D.   Ketorolac

6.   The oral equianalgesic dose for 4 mg of hydromorphone IV is approximately

   A.   2 mg PO

   B.   4 mg PO

   C.   10 mg PO

   D.   20 mg PO

7.   Convert hydromorphone 7.5 mg every 3 hours PO to sustained release morphine

   A.   240 mg PO BID every 12 hours

   B.   60 mg PO BID every 12 hours

   C.   120 mg PO BID every 12 hours

   D.   900 mg PO BID every 12 hours

8.   Convert morphine 10 mg SQ every 4 hours to the equianalgesic daily dose of long acting oxycodone (morphine 10 mg equals 20 mg oxycodone)

   A.   60 mg every 12 hours

   B.   40 mg every 12 hours

   C.   20 mg every 12 hours

   D.   10 mg every 12 hours

5. Answer is D

    A. Incorrect: Not available for parenteral use.

    B. Incorrect: Not available for parenteral use.

    C. Incorrect: Not available for parenteral use.

    D. **Correct:** Ketorolac is the only NSAID with a parenteral formulation available.

6. Answer is D

    A. Incorrect

    B. Incorrect

    C. Incorrect

    D. **Correct**: 4 mg current dose/1.5 mg current equivalent x 7.5 mg new equivalent = 20 mg new dose

7. Answer is C

    A. Incorrect

    B. Incorrect

    C. **Correct**: 7.5 mg x 8 = 60 mg 24-hour dose

        60 mg current dose/7.5 current equivalent x 30 mg new equivalent = 240 mg new dose

        240 mg/2 doses per day = 120 mg PO BID

    D. Incorrect

8. Answer is A

    A. **Correct**: 10 mg x 6 = 60 mg total daily dose

        60 mg current dose/10 mg current equivalent x 20 mg new equivalent = 120 mg new dose

        120 mg/2 doses per day = 60 mg every 12 hours

    B. Incorrect

    C. Incorrect

    D. Incorrect

9.   The most effective combination of drugs to relieve pain due to metastatic bone disease is

   A. Hydromorphone and diazepam

   B. Acetaminophen and lorazepam

   C. Morphine and acetaminophen

   D. Ibuprofen and morphine

10.   What is the starting dose of morphine in an opioid naïve patient experiencing dyspnea?

   A. 2.5 to 5 mg of oral morphine every 4 hours

   B. 60 mg of sustained release morphine every 12 hours

   C. 10 mg of SQ morphine every hour

   D. Morphine is not safe to use for dyspnea

11.   First line therapy for pneumocystis carinii pneumonia is most often

   A. Pentamidine

   B. Trimethoprim/sulfamethoxazole

   C. Dapsone

   D. Amphotericin B

9. Answer is D

   A. Incorrect: While hydromorphone would be effective as an opioid analgesic, the addition of diazepam, a benzodiazepine, would not provide additional benefit in the management of metastatic bone pain.

   B. Incorrect: Acetaminophen and lorazepam would provide minimum relief for metastatic bone pain.

   C. Incorrect: While morphine is an effective opioid analgesic like hydromorphone, acetaminophen is not as effective in metastatic bone pain as an NSAID.

   D. **Correct:** Morphine with ibuprofen combines the benefit of a centrally acting opioid with a peripherally acting NSAID. Ibuprofen is very effective as an adjuvant analgesic agent in combination with morphine for metastatic bone pain, enhancing the relief provided by the opioid without increasing the side effects.

10. Answer is A

    A. **Correct:** The opioid naive patient should be started on very low doses of oral morphine to assess the effectiveness without causing side effects or overdosing.

    B. Incorrect: Long acting morphine is not the drug of choice for dyspnea until effectiveness and dose have been appropriately titrated.

    C. Incorrect: Subcutaneous morphine is not necessary—it is more painful, invasive and inconvenient and has a variable absorption rate. It could be considered as an alternative in a patient that could not swallow.

    D. Incorrect: Morphine is very safe for dyspnea and in fact is the drug of choice.

11. Answer is B

    A. Incorrect: Pentamidine would be second line therapy if first line therapy failed.

    B. **Correct:** Trimethoprim/sulfamethoxazole is the first line therapy for pneumocystis carinii pneumonia treatment and is also used for prophylaxis.

    C. Incorrect: Dapsone is an alternative therapy but is not the preferred or commonly used agent.

    D. Incorrect: Amphotericin B is an antifungal agent given IV.

12. Mrs. Brown is currently receiving sustained release oxycodone 60 mg every 12 hours for metastatic breast carcinoma with metastasis to pelvis, spine, and left femur. She has taken 4 doses of oxycodone 20 mg over the past 24 hours for breakthrough pain. What is the new dose of sustained release oxycodone that should be initiated to relieve Mrs. Brown's pain?

   A. 65 mg

   B. 70 mg

   C. 75 mg

   D. 100 mg

13. Should the breakthrough dose for Mrs. Brown stay the same or increase?

14. Mr. Smith has multiple sites of bone metastases from his primary prostate carcinoma. He reports that despite taking sustained release oxycodone 30 mg every 12 hours, his pain level remains at "8" when ambulating. You notice he does not have any breakthrough pain prescriptions. In addition to adding an NSAID ATC, what dose of immediate release oxycodone would you expect his physician to order for breakthrough?

   A. 5 mg

   B. 10 mg

   C. 15 mg

   D. 20 mg

15. Maximum daily dose of megestrol acetate is

   A. 200 mg

   B. 400 mg

   C. 600 mg

   D. 800 mg

12. Answer is D

   A. Incorrect

   B. Incorrect

   C. Incorrect

   D. **Correct:** The daily dose of sustained release is 120 mg plus 80 mg of breakthrough is a total 24-hour dose of 200 mg, so the every 12-hours dose should be changed to 100 mg.

13. The breakthrough dose should be calculated as 10-15% of the 24-hour dose given every 1-2 hours PO as needed. 10-15% of 200 mg is 20-30 mg. The breakthrough dose could stay at 20 mg or be increased to 30 mg.

14. Answer is B

   A. Incorrect: Insufficient dose for breakthrough.

   B. **Correct:** Breakthrough dose should be 10-15 (up to 20) percent of the total daily dose given 1-2 hours PRN PO. That would be 6-9 mg (12 mg). Since his pain is significant when ambulating, the higher dose would be better and the 10 mg dose would be the most convenient.

   C. Incorrect: This dose would be more than is indicated.

   D. Incorrect: This dose would be more than is indicated.

15. Answer is D

   A. Incorrect: Megestrol acetate is normally given in doses of 400 mg BID.

   B. Incorrect: This is a one time dose of megestrol acetate—it is normally given 400 mg twice a day.

   C. Incorrect: Megestrol acetate can be given to a level of 800 mg a day.

   D. **Correct:** The maximum daily dose of megestrol acetate is 800 mg. It is normally prescribed as megestrol acetate 400 mg BID.

16. Medications that can color urine, feces, sputum, sweat, and tears a red-orange color and stain soft contact lenses are

   A. Dapsone and pentamidine

   B. Isoniazid and ethambutol

   C. Rifabutin and rifampin

   D. Azithromycin and clarithromycin

17. Which of the following pain medications must **NOT** be crushed?

   A. Morphine sulfate sustained release

   B. Acetaminophen with codeine

   C. Acetaminophen with oxycodone

   D. Acetaminophen with hydrocodone

18. A "ceiling dose" of a medication is

   A. The maximum safe dose to prevent respiratory depression

   B. The maximum dose giving therapeutic results without undesirable side effects

   C. The highest dose the pharmacy will dispense

   D. The highest dose in which the drug is manufactured

16.   Answer is C

   A. Incorrect: Dapsone is used to treat leprosy and pentamidine is used in the treatment of pneumocystis carinii pneumonia. Neither of these agents causes discolorations of bodily secretions.

   B. Incorrect: Although both of these agents treat pulmonary tuberculosis, neither causes discolorations of bodily secretions.

   C. **Correct:** These two antitubercular agents, or their metabolites, can permanently stain soft contact lenses and will discolor urine, feces, sputum, sweat, and tears.

   D. Incorrect: Both agents are macrolide antiinfectives but neither cause discoloration of bodily secretions.

17.   Answer is A

   A. **Correct:** Sustained release products become immediate release if crushed and may lead to overdosing.

   B. Incorrect: Acetaminophen with codeine can be crushed without loss of effect.

   C. Incorrect: Acetaminophen and oxycodone could be crushed without losing any effect.

   D. Incorrect: Acetaminophen and hydrocodone can be crushed without causing loss of effect.

18.   Answer is B

   A. Incorrect: Respiratory depression would be one but not the only undesirable side effect of a medication.

   B. **Correct:** Ceiling dose refers to the maximum dose giving therapeutic results without undesirable side effects.

   C. Incorrect: The pharmacy will dispense whatever dose the physician orders within the norm of that medication. If any discrepancies occur, the pharmacist is required to contact the physician for clarification.

   D. Incorrect: The ceiling dose is not the highest dose manufactured.

19.   For the patient with persistent pain from metastatic cancer, pain medications should be given

   A.   PRN to avoid addiction and tolerance

   B.   Four times daily

   C.   Via a patch or intravenously for more severe pain

   D.   Around the clock on a regular schedule; plus a PRN dose for breakthrough pain

20.   For patients placed on SR (sustained-release) opioids for chronic pain relief, which of the following drugs would be an appropriate choice for acute "breakthrough" pain?

   A.   Pentazocine

   B.   Hydromorphone

   C.   Butorphanol

   D.   Nalbuphine

21.   Which of the following opioid analgesics is usually **NOT** recommended in chronic pain due to the drug's short duration of action and toxic metabolites?

   A.   Meperidine

   B.   Morphine

   C.   Aspirin

   D.   Methadone

19.   Answer is D

   A. Incorrect: Patients experiencing persistent pain should always receive around the clock medications to assure a consistent blood level. PRN medications should be used for breakthrough pain.

   B. Incorrect: Administering pain medications four times a day may be insufficient to control pain around the clock especially if the scheduling is during the waking hours only. The schedule must match the recommended dosing interval of the drug as well. Some long acting preparations are scheduled less often and some short-acting medications more often.

   C. Incorrect: Patches and intravenous pain medication administration are justified only in specific situations. Around the clock oral opioids are the method of choice.

   D. **Correct:** The best method of managing pain control in the patient with persistent pain from metastatic cancer is to administer medications around the clock on a regular schedule and offer a PRN dose for breakthrough pain.

20.   Answer is B

   A. Incorrect: Pentazocine is an opioid agonist-antagonist and therefore may produce withdrawal symptoms if mixed with agonist opioids, has an analgesic ceiling and may have psychomimetic side effects.

   B. **Correct:** Hydromorphone is an opioid and very effective as a breakthrough analgesic with sustained release narcotics.

   C. Incorrect: Butorphanol is an opioid agonist-antagonist and therefore may produce withdrawal symptoms if mixed with pure agonist opioids. It has an analgesic ceiling and may have psychomimetic side effects.

   D. Incorrect: Nalbuphine is an opioid agonist-antagonist and therefore may produce withdrawal symptoms if mixed with pure agonist opioids. It has an analgesic ceiling and may have psychomimetic side effects.

21.   Answer is A

   A. **Correct:** Meperidine has a short duration of only two to three hours. Repeated doses may also lead to central nervous toxicity due to an accumulation of metabolites.

   B. Incorrect: Morphine is the opioid of choice for best analgesic response.

   C. Incorrect: Aspirin is not an opioid analgesic.

   D. Incorrect: Methadone has a long duration of action (6-8 hours) and an even longer half-life.

22. Neuropathic pain, which the patient might describe as burning, tingling, or shooting, would best be treated with which type of adjuvant analgesic?

A. Benzodiazepines

B. Nonsteroidal anti-inflammatory drug (NSAID)

C. Tricyclic antidepressant

D. Skeletal muscle relaxant

23. If the patient has a brain tumor and headache that may be caused from edema around the tumor, a useful medication to add to the current analgesic regime would be

A. Dexamethasone

B. Phenobarbital

C. Hydrochlorothiazide

D. Acetaminophen

24. The fentanyl transdermal patch is subcutaneously absorbed analgesia and

A. Is routinely changed every 72 hours

B. Absorbs better on skin over some adipose or muscle tissue

C. Can be changed every 48 hours if the patient consistently has increased pain on the third day

D. All of the above

22. Answer is C

    A. Incorrect: Neuropathic pain does not respond well to benzodiazepines.

    B. Incorrect: NSAIDs best relieve bone pain not neuritic type pain.

    C. **Correct:** Tricyclic antidepressants such as amitriptyline, doxepin, imipramine, and nortriptyline are the agents of choice in neuritic-type pain along with anticonvulsants.

    D. Incorrect: Skeletal muscle relaxants would best relieve muscle spasms not nerve pain.

23. Answer is A

    A. **Correct**: Cerebral edema is very responsive to corticosteroids. Dexamethasone produces beneficial effects within an hour of the dose administration.

    B. Incorrect: Phenobarbital is a barbiturate that depresses monosynaptic and polysynaptic transmission in the CNS and increases the threshold for seizure activity in the motor cortex.

    C. Incorrect: Hydrochlorothiazide is a thiazide diuretic that increases sodium and water excretion by inhibiting sodium and chloride reabsorption in the nephron's distal segment.

    D. Incorrect: Acetaminophen is thought to produce analgesia by inhibiting prostaglandin synthesis in the CNS but would have little to no benefit with cerebral edema.

24. Answer is D

    A. Incorrect: Normally the fentanyl patch should be changed every 72 hours. Other answers are also correct.

    B. Incorrect: Transdermal fentanyl does absorb better on skin over some adipose or muscle tissue. Other answers are correct also.

    C. Incorrect: The fentanyl patch can be changed every 48 hours if the patient consistently has pain on the third day. The other answers are also correct.

    D. **Correct:** The best answer for this question is all of the above.

25.	The drug of choice in addition to anticonvulsants for treating an active seizure in a terminally ill patient is

A.	Lorazepam

B.	Amitriptyline

C.	Prochlorperazine

D.	Prednisone

26.	The most appropriate drug for agitation associated with physical harm by the patient to self or others and/or psychotic tendencies is

A.	Prochlorperazine

B.	Morphine

C.	Haloperidol

D.	Dexamethasone

27.	All **EXCEPT** one of the following drugs are indicated to control nausea

A.	Prochlorperazine

B.	Dextroamphetamine

C.	Haloperidol

D.	Metoclopramide

25. Answer is A

   A. **Correct**: Lorazepam is a PRN order made available to treat an active seizure that occurs with a terminally ill patient who is currently being treated with anticonvulsants. Lorazepam can be given IV or sublingually using the Intensol solution.

   B. Incorrect: Amitriptyline is an antidepressant and would offer no benefit to seizure activity in the terminally ill.

   C. Incorrect: Prochlorperazine is an antiemetic and would offer no benefit and is contraindicated with CNS depression.

   D. Incorrect: Prednisone, as a corticosteroid, would offer no benefit in this situation.

26. Answer is C

   A. Incorrect: Prochlorperazine is an antiemetic contraindicated with those patients with CNS depression.

   B. Incorrect: Morphine is an opioid analgesic that offers little benefit for confusion and agitation unless the agitation is due to a pain syndrome.

   C. **Correct:** Haloperidol is an antipsychotic that blocks postsynaptic dopamine receptors in the brain. Recommended dose is 0.5–5 mg PO every 6–24 hours. Elderly patients usually require lower initial doses and a more gradual dosage titration.

   D. Incorrect: Dexamethasone is a corticosteroid recommended for treating cerebral edema and the prevention of seizure activity that may occur secondarily.

27. Answer is B

   A. Incorrect: Prochlorperazine is an antiemetic but so are haloperidol and metoclopramide

   B. **Correct**: Dextroamphetamine is a CNS stimulant.

   C. Incorrect: Haloperidol has antiemetic activity although it is primarily an antipsychotic agent.

   D. Incorrect: Metoclopramide is an antiemetic.

28. Intractable hiccups may be best treated with

A. Ondansetron

B. Phenytoin

C. Megestrol

D. Chlorpromazine

28.   Answer is D

   A. Incorrect: Ondansetron is a selective antagonist of a specific type of serotonin receptor located in the CNS and therefore is an antiemetic used to prevent nausea and vomiting associated with emetogenic chemotherapy.

   B. Incorrect: Phenytoin is an anticonvulsant that offers no benefit for intractable hiccups.

   C. Incorrect: Megestrol acetate is a progestin that changes a neoplastic tumor's hormonal environment thereby altering the neoplastic process. This mechanism does stimulate appetite but has no benefit for intractable hiccups.

   D. **Correct:** Chlorpromazine is one of the drugs of choice for intractable hiccups caused by stress to the diaphragm, which may be chemical, mechanical, or neurological. A dose of 25 mg PO or PR TID is recommended.

Conversions Worksheet

Formula for Converting to New Drug or New Route Using Equianalgesic Table (Appendix A):

$$\frac{\text{Current 24-hour dose}}{\text{Current equivalent \#}} \times \text{New equivalent \#} = \text{New 24-hour dose}$$

For Calculating Breakthrough Dose:

10-15% of 24-hour dose (can be up to 20%) available every 1-2 hour PRN orally

Problem 1: Mr. H is being switched by his doctor from PO hydromorphone to PO oxycodone. The patient is on 4 mg of hydromorphone every 4 hours. What will the patient's every 12 hour dose of oxycodone be? What should he have available for PRN?

What if you decided to schedule it every 8 hr instead?

Problem 2: Mrs. F has been on IV morphine, 4 mg/hour. She is now able to take oral meds and will be switched to oral morphine. What will her every 4 hourly dose be? What dose should she have for breakthrough pain?

What if the team decides to use transdermal fentanyl instead?

Conversions Worksheet Answers

Problem 1 Answer

4x6=24 Current dose equianalgesic #	÷	**7.5** Current drug	=	**3.2** Equianalgesic 24-hour dose	x	**20** New drug/ route equivalent #	=	**64 mg** New 24-hour dose units

64 ÷ 2 = 32 mg every 12 hours
for ease of administration 30 mg every 12 would be a good starting dose with adjustment in 24-48 hours upward depending on the number of breakthrough doses used (long acting oxycodone is available in 10, 20, and 40 mg tablets)

Breakthrough: 10%-15% of 24-hour dose (60 mg) for PRN = 6-9 mg or 5-10 mg every 1-2 hr PRN of immediate release oxycodone for ease of administration. If more than 3 doses of breakthrough medication are used in 24 hours, then the dose should be titrated upward

64 ÷ 3 = 21 every 8 hours
for ease of administration 20 mg long-acting oxycodone would be a good starting dose
Breakthrough would remain the same at 5-10 mg immediate release oxycodone every 1-2 hr PRN since it is calculated from the 24-hour dose (60 mg)

Problem 2 Answer

(4x24) = 96 ÷ 10 = 9.6 x 30 = 288
288 ÷ 6 = 48 mg every 4 hours of immediate release morphine or could be 145 mg of controlled release morphine every 12 hr or 90-100 mg every 8 hr.

10-15% for breakthrough = 28.8-43.2 of immediate release; for ease of administration 30-45 mg every 1-2 hr PRN immediate release morphine which is the same whether you are giving the controlled release every 12 hr or every 8 hr.

With these large doses orally, a change to a fentanyl patch should be considered; 50% of 288 would be 144 mcg/hr patch or one 100 mcg/hr patch and one 50 mcg/hr patch. The breakthrough dose could remain the same. Another way to calculate the breakthrough is 2% of the patch dose which would be 50 mg or, for ease of administration, 45 mg of immediate release morphine.

1/3

Problem 3: Mr. M is on oral meperidine 75 mg every 3 hours. He is having increased pain and it is anticipated he will not be able to tolerate side effects of increased meperidine. If he is switched to long-acting morphine, what would his 12-hourly dose be? What should his breakthrough dose be?

Problem 4: Mrs. D has been receiving hydromorphone 15 mg PO every 4 hours. Dr. B wants her switched to transdermal fentanyl because of her difficulty swallowing. What would you recommend for breakthrough pain?

What if the plan changes and the patient is to receive IV or SQ morphine instead? What would the hourly rate be?

Problem 5: A patient with significant, painful metastatic disease is being discharged from the hospital into hospice. He is currently receiving IV morphine 3 mg/hour plus has received 8 mg in additional boluses in the last 24 hours. What is the appropriate oral regimen that would provide equal analgesia?

Problem 3 Answer

$(75 \times 8) = 600 \div 300 = 2 \times 30 = 60$ $60 \div 2 = 30$ mg every 12 hours controlled release

10-15% for breakthrough = 6-9 mg or for ease of administration 5-10 mg every 1-2 hr PRN immediate release

Problem 4 Answer

$(15 \times 6) = 90 \div 7.5 = 12 \times 30 = 360$ mg 24-hour dose of morphine equivalent
50% or ½ of morphine equivalent = mcg/hr of transdermal fentanyl
180 mcg/hr, start with one 100 mcg/hr and one 75 mcg/hr transdermal patch

For breakthrough, recommend concentrated morphine solution, 20 mg/ml which can be administered sublingually. 10-15% of 360 mg = 36-54 mg every 1-2 hr PRN. For ease of administration, 2-3 ml sublingual PRN. Since this is a relatively large dose for sublingual, may want to consider SQ morphine PRN.
360 mg/30 x 10 = 120 mg 24-hour dose
10-15% = 12-18 mg SQ every 1-2 hr PRN or 10-15 mg SQ for ease of administration

If the plan changes to SQ or IV morphine around the clock, the calculation would be:

$(15 \times 6) = 90 \div 7.5 = 12 \times 10 = 120$ mg 24 hour dose = 5 mg/hr
Breakthrough dose would be 50-100% of the hourly rate, or 2.5-5 mg every 15-30 minutes PRN SQ/IV

Problem 5 Answer

Current 24-hour = 3 mg x 24 hours = 72mg
Breakthrough doses = 8 mg
Total 24-hour dose = 80 mg
80 mg/10 mg x 30 mg = 240 mg new 24-hour dose or 120 mg every 12 hours PRN of sustained release morphine
Breakthrough 10%-15% of 24° dose (240) = 24-36 mg every 1-2 hours which would be more easily dosed as 30 mg immediate release PRN

Problem 6: A patient has been taking 8 mg of hydromorphone every 4 hr PO and is now being converted to the new long acting hydromorphone. What will the every 12 hr dose be?

Problem 7: A patient needs to take 250 mg of long acting morphine every 12 hr PO. What brand name formulation of long acting morphine would be the easiest to dose?

Problem 6 Answer

Current 24 hour = 8 mg x 6 doses in 24 hours = 48 mg
Palladone™, the only long-acting formulation of hydromorphone currently available, comes in strengths of 12 mg, 16 mg, 24 mg, and 36 mg so the appropriate dose would be 24 mg every 12 hr PO.

Problem 7 Answer

Sustained release morphine is available generically and as MS Contin® SR in the following tablet strengths: 15 mg, 30 mg, 60 mg, 100 mg, 200 mg.

Oramorph® SR is available in 15 mg, 30 mg, 60 mg, and 100 mg tablets.

Extended release morphine is also available as Avinza® in 30 mg, 60 mg, 90 mg, and 120 mg strength capsules.

Kadian® is available in the United States in 20 mg, 30 mg, 50 mg, 60 mg, and 100 mg strength capsules.

Assuming equivalence of different preparations, using generic or MS Contin®, a dose of 260 mg or 230 mg could be given using only 2 tablets (200 mg + 30 mg or 60 mg).

Avinza® could be dosed in 2 tablets to provide 240 mg (120 mg + 120 mg).

An exact dose of 250 mg could be supplied using 3 capsules of Kadian® (100 mg x 2 + 50 mg).

Note:
When converting using equianalgesic tables and changing patients to an alternate opioid, keep in mind that each individual patient's response to a medication is unique, and it is better to be conservative to start unless you are changing drugs because the patient's pain is inadequately controlled. In other words, patients may not have the exact same tolerance to one opioid as to another. This is known as lack of complete cross tolerance. In general, it is recommended to start at a lower than equianalgesic dose when changing from one opioid to another.

Appendix A

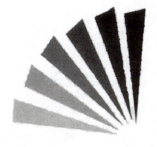

Opioid Dosing Equivalance

Drug	Dose (mg) Parenteral	Dose (mg) Oral	Duration (hours)
Morphine (IR)	10	30	3-4
Morphine, Controlled Release (MS Contin®, Oramorph SR®)	—	30	8-12
Hydromorphone (Dilaudid®)	1.5	7.5	3-4
Codeine	130	200	3-4
Oxycodone, Controlled Release (Oxycontin®)	—	20	8-12
Oxycodone (Roxicodone®, Percocet®)	—	20	3-4
Hydrocodone (Vicodin®, Lortab®)	—	30	3-4
Meperidine (Demerol®)	100	300+	2-3
Levorphanol (Levo-Dromoran®)	2	4	6-8
Methadone (Dolophine®)[,1]	10 acute pain 2-4 chronic pain		8
Fentanyl (Duragesic®, generic)	0.1	Convert present medication to 24 hour oral MS equivalent; then divide in half; this is mcg/hr dose of fentanyl	48-72
Propoxyphene (Darvon®; Darvocet®)	—	180	4

Important Note: If converting from one drug to another AND the patient's pain is well controlled, many experts recommend reducing the dose by 25% to account for incomplete cross tolerance. However, if you are converting from one drug to another AND the patient is in severe pain, dose reduction is often not necessary.

a. WARNING: Long-lived toxic metabolite; CNS stimulant, not recommended for long-term use

b. Methadone should be used with caution in older adults. Dose methadone using the following guidelines:[2-4]

 1. If the total morphine or equivalent dose per day is less than 90 mg (oral) a methadone ratio of 1:4 (methadone to morphine) is used. The total methadone dose is divided by 3 and given at 8-hour intervals.

 2. If the morphine or equivalent dose per day is between 90 and 300 mg (oral), a dose ratio of 1:8 (methadone to morphine) is used. The total methadone dose is divided by 3 and given at 8-hour intervals.

 3. If the morphine or equivalent dose per day is greater than 300 mg (oral), a dose ratio of 1:12 (methadone to morphine) is used. The total methadone dose is divided by 3 and given at 8-hour intervals.

 4. Patient maintained on an 8-hour schedule of methadone may have 10% of the daily dose for breakthrough pain

c. WARNING: Long-lived metabolite that is toxic to the central nervous system and cardiovascular system, not recommended for long-term use and use in the elderly.

Cited References

1. Paice JA, Fine P. Pain at the end of life. In: Ferrell B, Coyle N, eds. *Textbook of Palliative Nursing*. 2nd ed. New York, NY: Oxford University Press; 2006:131-154.

2. Miaskowski C, Cleary J, Burney R, Coyne P, Finley, R, Foster R, Grossman S, Janjan N, Ray J, Syrjala K, Weisman S, Zahrbock C. *Guideline for the Management of Cancer Pain in Adults and Children, APS Clinical Practice Guideline Series, No 3*. Glenview, IL: American Pain Society; 2005.

3. DeConno F, Groff L, Brunelle C, Zecca E, Ventafridda V, Ripamonit C. Clinical experience with oral methadone administration in the treatment of pain in 196 advanced cancer patients. *Journal of Clinical Oncology*. 1996;14:2836-2842.

4. Ripamonti C, Zecca E, Bruera E. An update on the clinical use of methadone for cancer pain. *Pain*. 1997;70:109-115.

GENERAL REFERENCES

Addington-Hall J.M, MacDonald LD Anderson HR. Randomized controlled trial of effects of coordinating care for terminally ill patients. *British Medical Journal*. 1992;305:1317-1322.

Administration on Aging, *Older population by age: 1900 to 2050*. Administration on Aging; 2000.

Alderman J. Fast Facts #96: Diarrhea in palliative care. End of Life Physician Education Resource Center. Available at www.eperc.mcw.edu/. Accessed August, 2003.

Allen JE. *Assisted Living Administration: The Knowledge Base*. New York, NY: Springer; 1999.

American Academy of Hospice and Palliative Medicine. *Position Statement: Comprehensive end-of-life care and physician-assisted suicide*. AAHPM. Available at: http://www.aahpm.org/positions/suicide.html. Accessed November 5, 2003.

American Cancer Society. Cancer facts and figures 2003: American Center Society. 2002.

American Health Care Association. *Facts and Trends: The Nursing Facility sourcebook*. Washington, DC; American Health Care Association, (AHCA); 1995.

American Medical Association. International Classification of Disease. Chicago, IL: AMA Press; 2001.

American Nurses Association. Position Statement: Active Euthanasia. *American Nurses Association, Task force on the Nurses' Role in End-of-Life Decisions, Center for Ethics and Human Rights* December 8, 1994. Available at: http://www.ana.org/readroom/position/ethics/eteuth.htm. Accessed July 16, 2004.

American Nurses Association. Position Statement: Assisted Suicide. *American Nurses Association, Task Force on the Nurse's Role in End-of-Life Decisions, Center for Ethics and Human Rights* December 8, 1994. Available at: http://www.ana.org/readroom/position/ethics/etsuic.htm. Accessed July 16, 2004.

American Nurses Association. *Code for nurses with interpretive statements*. Kansas City, MO: American Nurses Association; 1985.

American Nurses Association. *Scope and Standards of Advanced Practice Registered Nursing*. Washington, DC: American Nurses Association; 1996.

American Nurses Association. Code of ethics for nurses with interpretive statements. Washington, DC: American Nurses Association; 2001.

American Nurses Association. Position Statement: Promotion of Comfort and Relief of Pain in Dying Patients. American Nurses Association, Task Force on the Nurse's Role in End-of-Life Decisions. December 5, 2003. Available at: http://www.ana.org/readroom/position/ethics/etpain.htm. Accessed July 16, 2004.

American Pain Society. *Principles of Analgesic Use in the Treatment of Acute Pain and Cancer Pain*. 5th ed. Glenview, IL: Author; 2003.

American Society of Clinical Oncology Outcomes Working Group (ASCO), c.m., Outcomes of cancer treatment for technology assessment and cancer treatment guidelines. *Journal of Clinical Oncology*. 1995;14:671-679.

American Society of Pain Management Nurses. Position Statement on End of Life Care. *ASPMN*. Available at: http://www.aspmn.org/html/PSeolcare.htm. Accessed July 16, 2004.

American Society of Pain Management Nurses. *Position statement: Assisted suicide. ASPMN.* Available at: http://www.aspmn.org/html/PSassistsuicide.htm. Accessed July 16, 2004.

Bailey S. The concept of futility in healthcare decision making. *Nurs Ethics.* 2003;11(1):77-83.

Balanced Budget Act. In: *Congressional Record.* 1997.

Barilan YM. Revisiting the problem of Jewish bioethics: the case of terminal care. *Kennedy Institute of Ethics Journal.* 2003;13(2):141-168.

Barr JE. Principles of wound cleansing. *Ostomy/Wound Management.* 1995; 41(Supp 7A):15S-22S.

Baumrucker SJ. Current concepts in hospice care: Management of intestinal obstruction in hospice care. *The American Journal of Hospice and Palliative Care.* 1998;14(4):232-235.

Beauchamp TL, Childress JF. *Principles of Biomedical Ethics.* 5th ed. New York, NY: Oxford University Press; 2001.

Bednash G, Ferrell B. *End-of-Life Nursing Education Consortium (ELNEC).* Washington, DC: Association of Colleges of Nursing; 2006.

Benner P. *From Novice to Expert.* Menlo Park, CA: Addison-Wesley; 1984.

Benner P. The oncology clinical nurse specialist as expert coach. *Oncology Nursing Forum.* 1985;12(2):40-44.

Beresford L. The questions of growth. *Hospice.* 1995;6(4):24-26.

Bergstrom N, et al. *Pressure Ulcer Treatment: Clinical Practice Guideline. Quick Reference Guide for Clinicians, No. 15.* Rockville, MD; U.S. Department of Health and Human Services, Public Health Service, Agency for Health Care Policy and Research; 1994.

Blickensdorf L. Nurses and physicians: creating a collaborative environment. *Journal of IV Nursing,* 1996;19(3):127-131.

Born W, Greiner KA, Sylvia E, Butler J, Ahluwalia JS. Knowledge, attitudes, and beliefs about end-of-life care among inner-city African Americans and Latinos. [see comment]. *Journal of Palliative Medicine.* 2004;7(2):247-256.

Braveman P, Oliva G, Miller MG, Reiter R, Egerter S. Adverse outcomes and lack of health insurance among newborns in an eight-county area of California. *New England Journal of Medicine.* 1998;321:508-513.

Brenner R. Hospice care and palliative care: a perspective from experience. *The Hospice Journal.* 1999;14(3/4):155-166.

Brock DB, Foley DJ. Demography and epidemiology of dying in the U.S. with emphasis on deaths of older persons. *Hosp J.* 1998;13:49-60.

Brown G. *Statement before the IOM committee on care at the end of life on behalf of hospice of the Blue Grass.* In: *IOM Committee on Care at the End of Life.* Washington, DC; 1996.

Bruera E, Chadwick S, Brennis C. Methylphenidate associated with narcotic treatment of cancer pain. *Cancer Treatment Reports.* 1985;70:295-297.

Byock IR. *Dying Well: The Prospects for Growth at the End of Life.* New York, NY: Riverhead Books; 1997.

Byock IR. Hospice and palliative care: a parting of the ways or a path to the future. *Journal of Palliative Medicine.* 1998;1:165-176.

Calkin JD. A model for advanced nursing practice. *Journal of Nursing Administration.* 1984;14(1):24-30.

Callahan M, Kelley P. *Final Gifts: Understanding the Special Awareness, Needs and Communications of the Dying*. New York, NY: Bantam Books; 1993.

Campbell ML, Bizek KS, Thill M. Patient responses during rapid terminal weaning from mechanical ventilation: a prospective study. *Critical Care Medicine*. 1999;27(1):73-77.

Campbell T, Hately J. The management of nausea and vomiting in advanced cancer. *International Journal of Palliative Nursing*. 2000;6(1):18-20, 22-25.

Cantor MD, Braddock CH, 3rd, Derse AR, et al. Do-not-resuscitate orders and medical futility. *Archives of Internal Medicine*. 2003;163(22):2689-2694.

Cartwright J, Kayser-Jones J. End-of-life care in assisted living facilities: perceptions of residents, families and staffs. *Journal of Hospice and Palliative Nursing*. 2003;5(3):143-151.

Cassel C. *Letter to Colleagues about New Medicare Palliative Care Code*. New York, NY: Milbank Memorial Fund: 1996.

Center to Advance Palliative Care (CAPC). Availiable at http://www.capc.org/. Accessed April 24, 2005.

Chapin R, Dobbs-Kepper D. Aging in place in assisted living: philosophy versus policy. *The Gerontologist*. 2001;41(1):43-50.

Children's Hospice International. *Children's Hospice International: 2001 Informational Overview*. Alexandria, VA: Children's Hospice International; 2001.

Chochinov HM, Breitbart W. *Handbook of Psychiatry and Palliative Care*. New York, NY: Oxford University Press; 2000.

Clarfield AM, Gordon M, Markwell H, Alibhai SM. Ethical issues in end-of-life geriatric care: the approach of three monotheistic religions-Judaism, Catholicism, and Islam. *Journal of the American Geriatrics Society*. 2003;51(8):1149-1154.

Clark D, Neale B, Heather P. Contracting for palliative care. *Social Sciences and Medicine*. 1995;40(9):1193-1202.

Clark E. *Palliative Pain and Symptom Management for Children and Adolescents*. Alexandria, VA: Children's Hospice International and Division of Maternal and Child Health—U.S. Department of Health and Human Services: 1985.

Clauser SB. Recent innovations in home health care policy research. *Health Care Financing Review*. 1994;16(1):1-6.

Coda BA, O'Sullivan B, Donaldson G, Bohl S, Chapman CR, Shen DD. Comparative efficacy of patient-controlled administration of morphine, hydromorphone, or sufentanil for the treatment of oral mucositis pain following bone marrow transplantation (Abstract). *Pain*. 1997;72(3):333-346. Retrieved October 9, 2001 from the Ovid Bibliographic Records database.

Collins CA. Ascites. *Clinical Journal of Oncology Nursing*. 2001;5(1):43-44.

Conner SR. New initiatives transforming hospice care. *The Hospice Journal*, 1999;14(3/4):193-203.

Covinsky KE, Goldman L, Cook EF, Oye R, Desbiens N, Reding D, Fulkerson W, Connors AF Jr, Lynn J, Phillips RS. The impact of serious illness on patients' families. SUPPORT Investigators. Study to understand prognoses and preferences for outcomes and risks of treatment. Journal of the American Medical Association. 1994;272:1839-1844.

Crawley LM, Marshall PA, Lo B, Koenig BA. End-of-Life Care Consensus P. Strategies for culturally effective end-of-life care. *Annals of Internal Medicine*. 2002;136(9):673-679.

Cruzan v. Director of Missouri Department of Health. 397: DS 261; 1990.

deBlois J, O'Rourke KD. Issues at the end of life. the revised ethical and religious directives discuss suicide, euthanasia, and end-of-life procedures. *Health Progress.* 1995;76(8):24-27.

Dowdy MD, Robertson C, Bander JA. A study of proactive ethics consultation for critically and terminally ill patients with extended lengths of stay. *Critical Care Medicine.* 1998;26(2):252-259.

Doyle D, Hanks G, Cherny N, Calman K, eds. *Oxford Textbook of Palliative Medicine.* 3rd ed. New York, NY: Oxford University Press; 2004.

Emanuel EJ, Emanuel L. The economics of dying: the illusion of cost savings at the end of life. *New England Journal of Medicine.* 1994;330(8): 540-544.

Emanuel EJ, Fairclough DL, Slutsman J, Alpert H, Baldwin D, Emanuel LL. Assistance from family members, friends, paid care givers and volunteers in the care of terminally ill patients. New England Journal of Medicine. 1999;341(13):956-63.

Emanuel L, von Gunten C, Ferris F. *The education for physicians on end of life care (EPEC) curriculum.* Washington, DC: American Medical Association; 1999.

Erikson E. *Childhood and Society.* New York, NY: W.W. Norton & Co; 1963.

Ersek M. The continuing challenge of assisted death. *J Hospice and Palliative Nursing.* 2004;6(1):46-59.

Ewald R. Orphaned by AIDS. *Hospice.* 1995;6(5):28-32.

Fenton MV, Brykczynski KA. Qualitative distinctions and similarities in the practice of clinical nurse specialists and nurse practitioners. *Journal of Professional Nursing.* 1993;9:313-326.

Fenton MV. Identifying competencies of clinical nurse specialists. *Journal of Nursing Administration.* 1985;15(12):31-37.

Ferrell BR, Coyle N, eds. *Textbook of Palliative Nursing.* 2nd ed. New York, NY: Oxford University Press; 2006.

Ferrell BR, Juarez G, Borneman T. Outcomes of pain education in community home care. *Journal of Hospice and Palliative Nursing.* 1999;1(4):141-150.

Ferrell BR, Virani R, Grant M. Analysis of end-of-life content in nursing textbooks. *Oncology Nursing Forum.* 1999;26(5):869-876.

Ferris FD, Wodinsky HB, Kerr IG, Sone M, Hume S, Coons C. A cost-minimization study of cancer patients requiring a narcotic infusion in hospice and at home. *Journal of Clinical Epidemiology.* 1991;44(3):313-327.

Field MJ, Behrman RE. *When Children Die: Improving Palliative and End-of-Life Care for Children and their Families.* Washington, DC: National Academy Press; 2003.

Field MJ, Cassel CK. *Approaching death: improving care at the end of life.* Washington, DC: Institute of Medicine Task Force; 1997.

Foley KM, Gelband H, eds. *Improving Palliative Care for Cancer Summary and Recommendations.* Washington, DC: National Academy Press; 2001.

Foreman J. 70% would pick hospice. *The Boston Globe,* 1996;250(96)(October 4):A3.

Gornick M, McMillan A, Lubitz JA. A longitudinal perspective on patterns of Medicare payments. *Health Affairs.* 1996;12(2):140-150.

Grant M, et al. Assessment of quality of life with a single instrument. *Seminars in Oncology Nursing.* 1990;6(4):260-270.

Grant M, Ferrell BR, Rivera LM, Lee J. Unscheduled readmissions for uncontrolled symptoms: a health care challenge for nurses. Nursing Clinics of North America. 1995;30:673-682.

Hadley J, Steinberg EP, Feder J. Comparison of uninsured and privately insured hospital patients: Condition on admission, resource use and outcome. *Journal of the American Medical Association.* 1991;265(3):274-279.

Hamric AB. Spross JA, Hanson CM, eds. *Advanced Nursing Practice.* 2nd ed. Philadelphia, PA: W. B. Saunders Company; 2000:53-73.

Health Care Financing Administration (HCFA). *Transmittal #256: Medicare state operations manual.* Baltimore, MD: HCFA); 1994:Sections 2080-2087.

Health Care Financing Administration (HCFA). Trends in Medicare home health agency utilization and payment: Cys 1974-94. *Health Care Financing Review.* 1996;Statistical Suppl:76-77.

Holloran SD, Starkey GW, Burke PA, Steele G Jr, Forse RA. An educational intervention in the surgical intensive care unit to improve ethical decisions. Surgery. 1995;118(2):294-298.

Hospice and Palliative Nurses Association. HPNA Position Statement: Legalization of Assisted Suicide. 2006. Available at www.hpna.org/DisplayPage.aspx?Title=Position%20Statements. Accessed February 13, 2009.

Hospice and Palliative Nurses Association. *Position Statement: Providing Opioids at the End of Life.* Available at: http://www.hpna.org/positions.asp. Accessed July 16, 2004.

In re Quinlan. *755 A2A 647:* (New Jersey); 1976.

Innovations in End of Life Care. Project Safe Conduct Integrates Palliative Goals into Comprehensive Cancer Care, An Interview with Pitorak EF, Armour M. Available at: http://www2.edc.org/lastacts/archives/archivesJuly02/featureinn.asp Accessed April 24, 2005.

Jaakkimainen L, Goodwin PJ, Pater J, Warde P, Murray N, Rapp E. Counting the costs of chemotherapy in a National Cancer Institute of Canada randomized trial in non-small cell lung cancer. Journal of Clinical Oncology. 1990;8(8):1301-1309.

Jones DH. Caring for hospice patients in a long term care facility. *Caring Magazine.* 1993:228-230.

Joranson DE. Are health-care reimbursement policies a barrier to acute and cancer pain management? *Journal of Pain and Symptom Management.* 1994;9(4):244-253.

Kahn KL, Keeler EB, Sherwood MJ, Rogers WH, Draper D, Bentow SS, Reinisch EJ, Rubenstein LV, Kosecoff J, Brook RH. Comparing outcomes of care before and after implementation of the DRG-based prospective payment system. *Journal of the American Medical Association.* 1990; 264(15):1984-1988.

Keay TJ, Schonwetter RS. Hospice care in the long-term care facility. *American Family Physician.* 1998;56:491-494.

Kedziera P, Coyle N. Hydration, thirst and nutrition. In: Ferrell BR, Coyle N, eds. *Textbook of Palliative Nursing.* 2nd ed. New York, NY: Oxford University Press; 2006:239-248.

Kemp C. *Terminal Illness: A Guide to Nursing Care.* 2nd ed., Philadelphia, PA: Lippincott; 1999.

Kosecoff J, Kahn KL, Rogers WH, Reinisch EJ, Sherwood MJ, Rubenstein LV, Draper D, Roth CP, Chew C, Brook RH. Prospective payment system and impairment at discharge. The 'quicker-and-sicker' story revisited. *Journal of the American Medical Association.* 1990;264(15):1980-1983.

Krammer L, Muir C, Gooding-Gellar N, Williams M., von Gunten, C. Palliative care and oncology: Opportunities for nursing. *Oncology Nursing Update.* 1999;6:1-12.

Krammer LM, Ring AA, Martinez J, Jacobs MJ, Williams MB. The nurses' role in interdisciplinary and palliative care. In: Matzo ML, Sherman DW, eds. *Palliative Care Nursing: Quality Care to the End of Life.* New York, NY; Springer Publishing Co; 2001.

Kuebler KK, Berry PH, Hedirich DE. *End-Of-Life Care: Clinical Practice Guidelines.* Philadelphia, PA: WB Saunders; 2002.

Kuebler KK, Esper P, eds. *Palliative Practices from A-Z for the Bedside Clinician.* Pittsburgh, PA: Oncology Nursing Society; 2002.

Lagnado L. Rules are rules: Hospice's patients beat the odds, so Medicare decides to crack down. *The Wall Street Journal.* New York, NY. 2000:p. A1, A18.

LeChavlier T, Brisgand D, Douillard JY, Pujol JL, Alberola V, Monnier A, Riviere A, Lianes P, Chomy P, Cigolari S, et al. Randomized study of vinorelbine and cisplatin versus vindesine and cisplatin versus vinorelbine alone in advanced non-small cell lung cancer: results of a European multicenter trial including 612 patients. *Journal of Clinical Oncology.* 1994; 12(2):360-367.

Leonard DJ. Workplace education: adult education in a hospital staff development department. *Journal of Nursing Staff Development.* 1993;No 9:68-73.

Levetown M. Different—and needing to be more available. *Hospice.* 1995. 6(5):15-16, 36.

Levine C, ed. *Always on Call: When Illness Turns Families into Caregivers.* New York, NY: United Hospital Fund; 2004.

Levine C. Loneliness of the long-term caregiver. *N Engl J Med* 1999;340:1587-90.

Lewis L. Many-party harmony. *Hospice.* 1995;6(5): 8-9.

Lowenthal RM, Piaszczyk A, Arthur GE, O'Malley S. Home chemotherapy for cancer patients: cost analysis and safety. *Medical Journal of Australia.* 1996;165(4):184-187.

Luce JM, Alpers A. Legal aspects of withholding and withdrawing life support from critically ill patients in the United States and providing palliative care to them. *American Journal of Respiratory & Critical Care Medicine.* 2000;162(6):2029-2032.

Lynn J, Schuster JL, Kabcenell A. *Improving Care for the End of Life: A Sourcebook for Health Care Managers and Clinicians.* New York, NY: Oxford University Press; 2000.

Manning WG, Newhouse JP, Duan N, Keeler EB, Leibowitz A, Marquis MS. Health insurance and the demand for medical care: Evidence from a randomized experiment. *American Economic Review.* 1987;77(3):251-277.

Matzo ML, Sherman DW. *Gerontologic Palliative Care Nursing.* St. Louis, MO; CV Mosby; 2004.

Matzo M, Sherman D, eds. *Palliative Care Nursing: Quality Care to the End of Life.* New York, NY: Springer Publishing Company; 2001.

McCaffery M, Pasero C. *Pain: Clinical Manual.* St. Louis, MO: Mosby; 1999.

Miaskowski C, Cleary J, Burney R, Coyne P, Finley R, Foster R, Grossman S, Janjan N, Ray J, Syrjala K, Weisman S, Zahrbock C. Guidelines for the management of cancer pain in adults and children. *APS Clinical Practice Guidelines Series.* No 3. Glenview, IL: American Pain Society; 2005.

Miller SC, Gozalo P, Mor V. Hospice enrollment and hospitalization of dying nursing home patients. *American Journal of Medicine.* 2001;111(1):38-44.

Millman M. *Access to Health Care in America.* Washington, DC: Institute of Medicine—National Academy Press; 1993.

Morita T, Tsunoda J, Inoue S, Chihara S. Effects of high dose opioids and sedatives on survival in terminally ill cancer patients. *Journal of Pain & Symptom Management.* 2001;21(4):282-289.

Nation RL, Evans AM, Milne RW. Pharmacokinetic drug interactions with phenytoin (Part I). *Clinical Pharmacokinetics.* 1997;18(1):37-60.

National Center for Assisted Living (NCAL). Assisted living resident profile. 2001. Available at http://www.ncal.org/about/resident.htm. Accessed June 19, 2004.

National Consensus Project for Quality Palliative Care. Clinical Practice Guidelines for Quality Palliative Care. Pittsburgh, PA: National Consensus Project for Quality Palliative Care; 2004:18. Available at www.nationalconsensusproject.org. Accessed July 29, 2004.

National Hospice and Palliative Care Organization. *Facts and Figures 2003.* Arlington, VA: National Hospice and Palliative Care Organization; 2004.

National Hospice and Palliative Care Organization. *Hospice fact sheet.* Alexandria, VA: National Hospice and Palliative Care Organization; 2000.

National Hospice and Palliative Care Organization. NHPCO *Facts and figures (Updated February 2004),* National Hospice and Palliative Care Organization; 2004.

National Hospice and Palliative Care Organization. *Press release: New findings address escalating end-of-life debate.* Alexandria, VA: National Hospice and Palliative Care Organization; 1996.

National Hospice and Palliative Care Organization. *Statement of the national hospice organization opposing the legalization of euthanasia and assisted suicide*: NHPCO; 1999.

National Hospice Organization. *A Pathway for Patients and Families Facing Terminal Illness.* Arlington, VA: National Hospice Organization; 1997:5-6.

Natural Death Act. *Washington State.* Vol RCW 70.122.010; 1992.

Naylor MD, Brooten D, Campbell R, Jacobsen BS, Mezey MD, Pauly MV, Schwartz JS. Comprehensive discharge planning and home follow-up of hospitalized elders. A randomized clinical trial. Journal of the American Medical Association. 1999;281:613-620.

Newhouse JP, Group IE. *Free for all? Lessons from the Rand Health Insurance Experiment.* Cambridge, MA: Harvard University Press; 1993.

O'Connor P. Clinical paradigm for exploring spiritual concerns. In Doka KJ, Morgan J, eds. *Death and Spirituality,* New York, NY: Baywood Publishing Company; 1993.

O'Connor P. Hospice vs. palliative care. *The Hospice Journal.* 1999;14(3/4):123-137.

Oregon Nurses Association. ONA provides guidance on nurses' dilemma. *Oregon Nurses Assoc.* Available at: http://www.oregonrn.org/associations/3019/files/AssistedSuicide.pdf. Accessed July 19, 2004.

Paice JA. *Neurological disturbances.* In: Ferrell BR, Coyle N, eds. *Textbook of Palliative Nursing.* 2nd ed. New York, NY: Oxford University Press; 2006:365-374.

Panke J, Coyne P, eds. *Conversations in Palliative Care.* Pensacola, FL: Pohl Publishing; 2004:41-57.

Pauls M, Hutchinson RC. Bioethics for clinicians: 28. Protestant bioethics. *Canad Med Assoc J.* 2002;166(3):339-343.

Payne SK. *A High Volume Specialist Palliative Care Unit (PCU) and Team Reduces End of Life (EOL) Costs.* 2001 ASCO Annual Meeting. American Society of Clinical Oncology.

Petrillo M, Sanger S. *Emotional Care of Hospitalized Children: An Environmental Approach*. 2nd ed. Philadelphia, PA: J.B. Lippincott; 1980.

Pioneer Programs in Palliative Care: Nine Case Studies. New York, NY:Milbank Memorial Fund; 2000. The Center to Advance Palliative Care, 2005.

Portenoy PR. Defining Palliative Care. Newsletter, Dept. of Pain and Palliative Care—Beth Israel Medical Center; 1998.

PPRC, P.P.R.C. *Annual Report to Congress*. Washington, DC: PPRC, Physician Payment Review Commission; 1993.

Preston FA, Cunningham RS. *Clinical Guidelines for Symptom Management in Oncology: A Handbook for Advanced Practice Nurses*. New York, NY: Clinical Insights Press; 1998.

Puntillo K, Stannard D. The intensive care unit. In: Ferrell B, Coyle N, eds. *Textbook of Palliative Nursing*. 2nd ed. New York, NY: Oxford University Press: 2006:817-834.

Raftery JP, Addington-Hall JM, MacDonald LD, Anderson HR, Bland JM, Chamberlain J, Freeling P. A randomized controlled trial of the cost-effectiveness of a district co-coordinating service for terminally ill cancer patients. *Palliative Medicine*. 1996;10:151-161.

Rando TA. *Grief, Dying and Death: Clinical Interventions for Caregivers*. Champaign, IL: Research Press; 1984.

Rich MW, Beckham V, Wittenberg C, Leven CL, Freedland KE, Carney RM. A multidisciplinary intervention to prevent the readmission of elderly patients with congestive heart failure. The New England Journal of Medicine. 1995;333(18):1190-1195.

Rogers B. When young life is lost. *Hospice*. 1995;6(5):24-27.

Rosenberg HM, Ventura SJ, Maurer JD. *Births and Deaths United States, 1995*. Monthly Vital Statistics Report, Preliminary Data from the Centers for Disease Control and Prevention, National Center for Health Statistics; 1996.

Rousseau P. Nonpain symptom management in terminal care. *Clinics in Geriatric Medicine*. 1996;12(2):313-327.

Rubenstein LV, Kahn KL, Reinisch EJ, Sherwood MJ, Rogers WH, Kamberg C, Draper D, Brook RH. Changes in quality of care for five diseases measured by implicit review, 1981-1986. *Journal of the American Medical Association*. 1990;264(15):1974-1979.

Ryndes T, et al. *Just Access and Human Values in Hospice and Palliative Care: Building an End-of-Life Care System for the 21st Century*. The Hastings Center and the National Hospice Work Group. 2001

Saunders C. Forward. In: Doyle D, Hanks G, MacDonald N, eds. *Oxford Textbook of Palliative Care*. New York, NY: Oxford University Press; 1993.

Scanlon C. Assisted suicide: clinical realities and ethical challenges. *American Journal of Critical Care*. 1996;5(6):397-403; quiz 404-395.

Scanlon C. Defining standards for end-of-life care. *American Journal of Nursing*, 1997;97(11):58-60.

Scanlon C. Ethical concerns in end-of-life care. *American Journal of Nursing*. 2003;103(1):48-55; quiz 56.

Schneiderman LJ, Gilmer T, Teetzel HD, et al. Effect of ethics consultations on nonbeneficial life-sustaining treatments in the intensive care setting: a randomized controlled trial. *JAMA*. 2003;290(9):1166-1172.

Shafazand S, Crawley LM, Raffin T, Koenig B. Withholding and withdrawing treatment: the doctor-patient relationship and the changing goals of care. In: Beger A, Portenoy R, Weissman D, eds. *Principle and*

Practice of Palliative Care and Supportive Oncology. 2nd ed. Philadelphia, PA: Lippincott Williams & Wilkins; 2002:880-890.

Shuler PA, Davis JE. The Shuler nurse practitioner practice model: a theoretical framework for nurse practitioner clinicians, educators and researchers. Part I. *Journal of the American Academy of Nurse Practitioners*. 1993;5:11-18.

Smith SA, ed. *Hospice and Palliative Care Clinical Practice Monograph: Treatment of End-Stage Non-Cancer Diagnoses*. Dubuque, IA: Kendall/Hunt Publishing Co.; 2001.

Smith TJ, Hillner BE, Neighbors DM, McSorley PA, Le Chevalier T. An economic evaluation of a randomized clinical trial comparing vinorelbine, vinorelbine plus cisplatin and vindesine plus cisplatin for non-small cell lung cancer. *Journal of Clinical Oncology*. 1995;13(9):6-2173.

Snow C. New hospice horizons: HMO expansion could boost provider's popularity. *Modern Healthcare*. 1997;27(9):90, 92.

Soumerai SB, Ross-Degnan D, Avorn J, McLaughlin T, Choodnovskiy I. Effects of Medicaid drug-payment limits on admission to hospitals and nursing homes. *New England Journal of Medicine*. 1991;325(15):1072-1077.

Souquet PJ, Chauvin F, Boissel JP, Cellerino R, Cormier Y, Ganz PA, Kaasa S, Pater JL, Quoix E, Rapp E, et al. Polychemotherapy in advanced non-small cell lung cancer: a meta-analysis. Lancet. 1993;342: 19-21.

Standards and Accreditation Committee, Medical Guidelines Task Force. Medical Guidelines for Determining Prognosis in Selected Non-Cancer Disease. 2nd ed. Arlington, VA: National Hospice and Palliative Care Organization; 1996.

Stanley K, Zoloth-Dorfman L. Ethical considerations. In: Ferrell B, Coyle N, eds. *Textbook of Palliative Nursing*. 2nd ed. New York: Oxford University Press; 2006:1031-1054.

Stuck AE, Aronow HU, Steiner A, Alessi CA, Bula CJ, Gold MN, Yuhas KE, Nisenbaum R, Rubenstein LZ, Beck JC. A trial of annual in-home comprehensive geriatric assessments for elderly people living in the community. The New England Journal of Medicine. 1995;333(18):1184-1189.

Sulmasy DP. *The Healer's Calling*. New York, NY/Mahway: Paulist Press; 1997.

SUPPORT, A controlled trial to improve care for seriously ill hospitalized patients: a study to understand prognoses and preferences for outcomes and risks of treatments (SUPPORT). *Journal of the American Medical Association*. 1995;274:1951-1598.

Swan JH, Dewit S, Harrington C. *State Medicaid Reimbursement Methods and Rates for Nursing Homes*. Wichita, KS: Wichita State University; 1994.

Sykes N, Thorns A. The use of opioids and sedatives at the end of life. *Lancet Oncology*. 2003;4(5):312-318.

Taber CW. *Taber's Cyclopedic Medical Dictionary*. 20th ed. Philadelphia, PA: A. Davis; 2005.

Teno J, Byock IR, Field MJ. Research agenda for developing measures to examine quality of care and quality of life of patients diagnosed with life limiting illness. *Journal of Pain and Symptom Management*. 1999;17(2):75-82.

Teno JM, Casey VA, Welch LC, Edgman-Levitan S. Patient-focused, family-centered end-of-life medical care: views of the guidelines and bereaved family members. *Journal of Pain Symptom Management*. 2001;22:738-51.

Teno JM, Weitzen S, Wetle T, Mor V. *Persistent Pain in Nursing Home Residents*. JAMA. 2001;285:2081.

The Dartmouth Atlas of Health Care. 1999. Available at http://www.dartmouthatlas.org/atlaslinks/99atlas.php. Accessed April 18, 2005.

Thomasma DC. An analysis of arguments for and against euthanasia and assisted suicide: Part one. *Cambridge Quarterly of Healthcare Ethics*. 1996;5(1):62-76.

Thomasma DC. Assessing the arguments for and against euthanasia and assisted suicide: Part Two. *Cambridge Quarterly of Healthcare Ethics*. 1998;7(4):388-401.

U.S. Department of Health and Human Services. *2003 CMS statistics*. Available at: http://www.cms.hhs.gov/researchers/pubs/03cmsstats.pdf.

Ventura SJ, et al. *Births and Deaths: Preliminary Data for 1997*. Hyattsville: National Center for Health Statistics; 1998.

von Gunten C, Muir C. Fast Facts #45: Medical management of bowel obstruction. End of Life Physician Education Resource Center. Availiable at www.eperc.mcw.edu/. Accesed July, 2001.

Wadsworth B. *Piaget's Theory of Cognitive Development*. New York, NY: David McKay Co; 1971.

Waller A, Caroline NL. *Handbook of palliative care in cancer*. 2nd ed. Boston, MA: Butterworth-Heinemann; 2000.

Walsh T, Rivera N, Kaiko R. Oral morphine and respiratory function amongst hospice inpatients with advanced cancer. *Support Care Cancer*. 2003;11(12):780-784.

Walsh TD. Opiates and respiratory function in advanced cancer. *Recent Results in Cancer Research*. 1984;89:115-117.

Way J, Back AL, Curtis JR. Withdrawing life support and resolution of conflict with families. *BMJ*. 2002;325(7376):1342-1345.

Weeks WB, Kofoed LL, Wallace AE, Welch HG. Advance directives and the cost of terminal hospitalization. *Archives of Internal Medicine*. 1994; 154(18):2077-2083.

Weissert WG, A new policy agenda for home care. *Health Affairs*. 1991; 10(2):67-77.

Weissman D. Fast Facts #1: Treating terminal delirium. End of Life Physician Education Resource Center. Availiable at www.eperc.mcw.edu/. Accessed May, 2000.

Weissman DE, Ambuel B, Hallenback J. Improving end-of-life care: a resource guide for physician education. Medical College of Wisconsin. 2000:50.

West SK, Levi L. Culturally appropriate end-of-life care for the Black American. *Home Healthcare Nurse*. 2004;22(3):164-168.

Wilson RK, Weissman D. Fast Facts #57: Neuroexcitatory effects of opioids: Patient assessment. End of Life Physician Education Resource Center. Available at www.eperc.mcw.edu/. Accessed December, 2001.

Wilson WC, Smedira NG, Fink C, McDowell JA, Luce JM. Ordering and administration of sedatives and analgesics during the withholding and withdrawal of life support from critically ill patients. *JAMA*. 1992;267(7):949-953.

Wodinsky HB, DeAngelis C, Rusthoven JJ, Kerr IG, Sutherland D, Iscoe N, Buckman R, Kornijenko M. Re-evaluating the cost of outpatient cancer chemotherapy. *Canadian Medical Association Journal*. 1987;137(10):903-906.

Wong DL. *Wong & Whaley's Clinical Manual of Pediatric Nursing*. 5th ed. St. Louis, MO: Mosby; 2000.

Worden JW. *Children and Grief: When a Parent Dies*. New York, NY: The Guilford Press; 1996.

Worden JW. *Grief Counseling and Grief Therapy*. 2nd ed. New York, NY: Springer; 1991.

World Health Organization. *National Cancer Control Programs: Policies and Managerial Guidelines*. 2nd ed. Author: 2002.

Yarbro CH, Frogge MH, Goodman M. Cancer Nursing: Principles and Practice. 6th ed. Sudbury, MA: Jones and Bartlett; 2005.

Yates P, Stetz KM. Families' awareness of and response to dying. *Oncology Nursing Forum*. 1999;26(1):113-120.

Zerzan J, Stearns S, Hanson L. Access to palliative care and hospice in nursing homes. *Journal of the American Medical Association*. 2000;284(10):2489-2493.